Pediatric Pedorthics 101

For

KID'S

FEET

Inna Chon, Certified Pedorthist

Pediatric Pedorthics 101, For Kid's Feet

Copyright © 2022 by Inna Chon

First Published: 2022, United States of America

Revised: 2025

Publisher: Feet Balance Orthotics LLC

LCCN: 2022900751

ISBN: 978-1-947142-09-1 (paperback, black & white)
ISBN: 978-1-947142-05-3 (paperback, full color)
ISBN: 978-1-947142-06-0 (eBook)

Illustrations by Inna Chon

Cover and interior design by Inna Chon

Preface

When I discovered that the small joints on top of the foot—the ones that form the arch—falling with each step, I was literally shocked. I knew there were joints in our foot, but I had never thought how they relate to our body weight, posture, and the alignment of our entire body structure.

At that time, I was working as an animator at Disney Feature Animation Studio in Burbank, California. While analyzing foot structure, its mechanics, walking cycle with weight and ground reaction force, I could tell the Tarsal joint—a group of small joints that forms the arch, yet unknown to most people—needs support from under to keep the joint from falling.

When tarsal joint falls, the entire foot bones go out of alignment, including the anklebone. Tilted anklebones throw our entire body structure out of alignment from the feet up. A body standing out of alignment cannot develop its full strength and cannot use its full range of motion, and this surely damages the foot and major joints as well.

This tarsal joint starts to fall when toddlers start learning to stand and walk. That means our body is growing up and living out of alignment since we are toddlers, setting the stage for numerous foot and major joint issues, such as flat feet, bow legs, knock knees, scoliosis—just to name a few—and eventually arthritis in the feet and major joints.

We all know when foundation goes off; the entire structure goes out of alignment, causing many mechanical problems. When tarsal joint falls, we have to deal with biomechanical issues—a lot more complicated problems than just mechanical problems—that most people are suffering from. Yet, no one seems to realize the root cause of those problems is the fallen tarsal joint that tilts the anklebone.

Once we understand the foot structure, and how our body weight falls on it, we all can clearly see how these problems stem from the fallen tarsal joint— because it's really not rocket science. It's just like analyzing issues in a car running with tilted wheels. How has such an obvious and important fact been hiding in plain sight for centuries..?!

I began sharing my discovery with healthcare professionals whenever I had the opportunity. But soon, I realized they were not interested in hearing me, without a U.S medical credential, talking about the root cause of all those complicated foot and major joints problems. I needed proper credentials to be taken seriously.

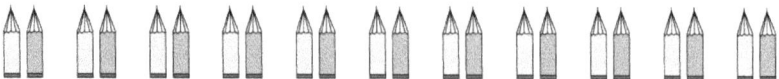

My Credentials

Then I learned about Pedorthists—medical professionals providing orthotics and footwear for foot health. How perfect the title is..!! "Ped-" means the foot, "-orthist" means one who aligns. I became a Certified Pedorthist (C-Ped) in 2005 after attaining my pedorthic credential at the Foot & Ankle Institute of Temple University in Philadelphia, Pennsylvania.

Soon, I realized the Pedorthic field lacked a reliable test to check if the foot bones are properly aligned or not. That inspired me to developed a test with a hypothesis of a simple logic of basic law of physic:

"A body stands out of alignment cannot use its full strength and full range of motion. But a body stands in alignment can use its full strength and full range of motion."

It's a simple theory, but when this law of physics is violated, we cannot avoid physical problems. I named the test the **"Anklebone Alignment Test,"** because the anklebones are the ones to determine whether the feet and the rest of the body are functioning in alignment or not.

As an animator, I know how to analyze movement with weight and ground reaction force—the foot has to deal with each step, and developed keen eyes for subtle movements. Animators have to catch any unnatural movement, especially, in slow motions, even less than 0.3mm mechanical pencil's lead thickness can cause wobbling in the movements.

When that happens, the problematic drawings have to be located, and those inconsistent line thicknesses have to be adjusted with sharp edged erasers—which I enjoyed doing that. With this skill, I could see that on tilted anklebones, our body compensating constantly with subtle movements.

And I studied physical therapy at Korea Medical College in South Korea that helps me to understand how aligning anklebones eliminates the root cause of foot and major joint problems, and our society in need of many pedorthists to align people's tilted anklebones—at every corner of the streets.

Lastly, while working for Disney, I took evening courses in fashion design at the Fashion Institute of Design and Merchandising (FIDM) in Los Angeles, California. I enjoy designing clothes. With this, I can foresee that orthotics may soon become a sought-after fashion item—much like eyeglasses.

My hope is that this book helps people to realize the importance of aligning our children's anklebones, so their bodies can grow and function in alignment—preventing many problems in the feet and major joint down the road.

Table of Contents

Introduction

"Mom, look at my flat feet..!! My tarsal joints are collapsed, completely..!!"

"Dad..! I need Orthotics! My Tarsal Joints are Falling and my Feet are Not Balanced..!!!"

"Ugh, I fell again..! Hate my tilted anklebones..! My body is so out of balance, Can't you see, mom? Get me orthotics, please..!!!"

Of course, your toddlers aren't able to describe collapsing of their tarsal joint—most people never heard of—like above. But they are expressing it with their feet, and the way they stand and walk. Yes, that's how toddlers start dealing with harsh reality; those flat floors do not conform to their feet with the arches at the bottom, and no one pays attention to it.

You might think that kids' having flat feet is normal, and it's cute when that little plump body wobbles and falls as they venture out to stand and walk. But once you understand how kid's foot bones grow while their entire body weight falling on their developing tarsal joint on top of their foot, it will begin to dawn on you that kids' having flat feet is not normal, and wobbly standing, staggering, and falling are not cute things anymore . . . they are rather cruel things, because of our ignorance, they are trying to stand and walk with all the foot bones out of alignment.

1

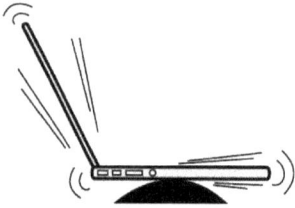

You wouldn't use a flat-bottomed computer on a rounded surface as it fluctuates and shakes all the time; it would not be efficient to use, and could damage the computer's hardware, and may even mess up the software down the road. A flat-bottomed object should be placed on flat surface for balance and stability.

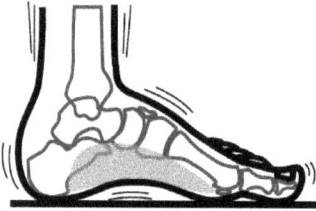

Likewise, our foot with an arch at the bottom should not stand or walk on flat surfaces, because the tarsal joint in the arch will fluctuate and shake all the time—as it falls with each step; this will stress our body not only physically (hardware) but mentally (software) also. Yet, we are doing this to our own "body machine" that would not be replaced since we were toddlers.

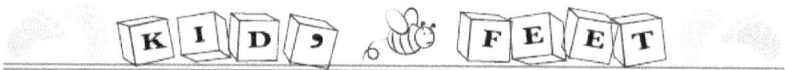

KID'S FEET

Chapter 1

Foot, the Foundation

When we think about the foot, we need to think about weight. The foot, the foundation of our body, at the bottom of our body, has to carry our entire body weight. Our small, yet, intricately designed foot with so many joints has a specific way to handle the weight. If we don't use our feet properly for their weight-bearing function, the feet will have problem, so will the rest of our body.

A typical 1-year-old weighs 20 pounds, while their foot weighs less than 1 pound. By age 18, the average body weight is around 120 pounds, and each foot weighs around 2 pounds. In other words, while Body weight multiples 6 times, each foot weight only doubles. That's it. When we gain weight, it sits above the feet.

Teenagers take about 10,000 steps a day (some more, some less), just like adults. Even someone who walks only 5,000 steps a day, each foot has to handle 2,500 times of the shock that is generated by its entire body weight—plus whatever they are carrying—on flat, hard floors. On top of all that, most kids are in mood of running and jumping. That multiplies the impact on their foot 3-4 times of their body weight.

The important thing is keeping our foot bones in alignment while we are on our feet, doing whatever. We don't want our feet carrying our body with all the foot bones out of alignment. But that's exactly what's happening, since babies begin to stand and take their first step. We need to make sure their foot bones are working in alignment. How..? With orthotics. Orthotics are not just for people with some foot or other issues. They are the essential devise for the alignment of our body from the feet up. Basically, for our body's overall health. Really..?

Yes, understanding the full-grown foot structure can help us to see why our feet need orthotics.

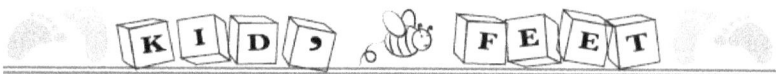

Foot Bone Structure

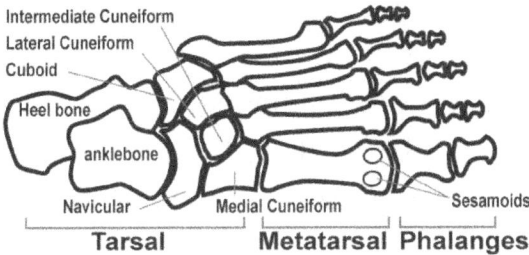

Intermediate Cuneiform
Lateral Cuneiform
Cuboid
Heel bone
anklebone
Navicular   Medial Cuneiform   Sesamoids
Tarsal   Metatarsal   Phalanges

There are 28 bones per foot: the oddly shaped 7 tarsal bones, 5 metatarsal bones of similar shape, except the 5th metatarsal bone that connects to the pinky toe having wider root area, and 2 tiny oval-shaped sesamoids under the 1st metatarsal head. All of these 14 bones form the arch. Front of the metatarsal heads—the front of the arch—are 14 toe bones (the phalanges, mini version of metatarsal bones) forming the 5 toes. The big toe made with 2 bones and 4 small toes with 3 bones

This foot structure can be divided into 2 parts: the arch and the toes, like below illustration.

Top View	Medial View	Lateral View

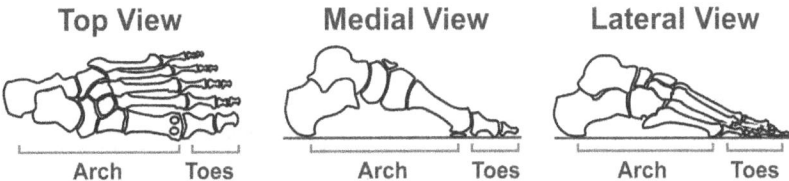

Arch	Toes	Arch	Toes	Arch	Toes

Each part shares the same number of bones. 14 for the arch, 14 for the toes—easy to remember. But the volume is quite different. It's about 80 to 20 ratio. The arch makes up about 80% of the foot, and 5 toes about 20% of the foot. Actually, when you look at the foot, the whole foot is the arch, except those five toes.

Also, notice that all of the foot bones are arranged horizontally, in a side-by-side manner, except the anklebone sits askew to the medial side over the heel bone and 2 sesamoids under the 1st metatarsal head.

This arrangement is quite opposite from the other weight-bearing joints above the anklebone that are standing vertically on top of each other.

Tarsal Joint

Have you ever heard of the tarsal joint? The tarsal joint is located on top of the foot and forms the arch in our foot, and it is the most complicated joint in our body. Despite the name, it's not a single joint. It's a group of small joints, having whopping 21 tiny joints.

Tarsal Joint

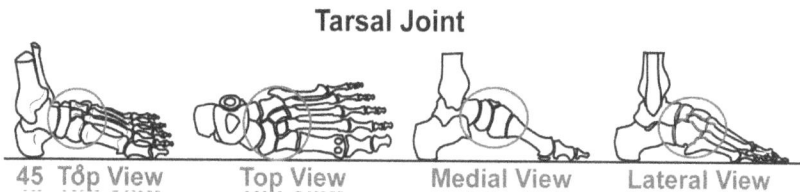

45 Top View   Top View   Medial View   Lateral View

The tarsal joint is constructed with those 7 tarsal bones and 5 metatarsal bones (altogether 12 bones), and they are arranged like a 3D puzzle, and the anklebone (talus) is one of the 7 tarsal bones on which the leg bone stands. (Just notice the 2 sesamoids under the 1st metatarsal head are part of the arch, but not part of the tarsal joint).

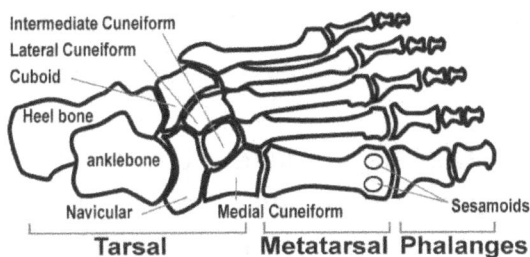

Intermediate Cuneiform
Lateral Cuneiform
Cuboid
Heel bone
anklebone
Navicular
Medial Cuneiform
Sesamoids

Tarsal   **Metatarsal Phalanges**

This illustration with the names of the bones in the tarsal joint shows the shape of each bones in the tarsal joint from the top.

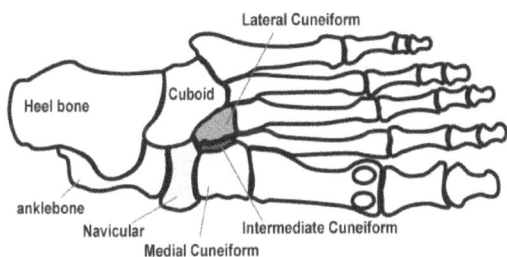

Lateral Cuneiform
Cuboid
Heel bone
anklebone
Navicular
Medial Cuneiform
Intermediate Cuneiform

This one shows the bottom shape of each bones in the tarsal joint. They look quite different from the top. The bottom of the cuboid, medial cuneiform, and heel bone are wider than their top, while the bottoms of the navicular, intermediate cuneiform, and lateral cuneiform are narrower than their top. This is how the tarsal joint is interlocked like a complex 3D puzzle.

Look at the bottoms of the intermediate and lateral cuneiforms that are situated at the middle top of the arch. Especially, the intermediate cuneiform—the darkest peekaboo bone where the second toe connects—has the narrowest bottom, forming a wedge shape. These two bones are locked in place, flanked by the medial cuneiform and cuboid with wide bottoms.

This interlocking arrangement makes it difficult for the tarsal joint to become disengaged. The complexity of this joint is hard to understand in just 2-dimensions. If you like to have a hands-on understanding, you can examine yourself with a real foot bone model. While examining, see how our body weight falls and transfers through this tarsal joint to get the glimpse of how these small joints handle our body weight. Then you might understand why this tarsal joint needs support from under to keep this joint from falling—from its tiny range of motion.

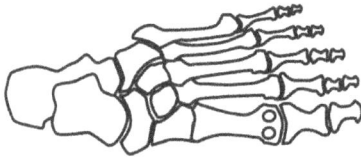 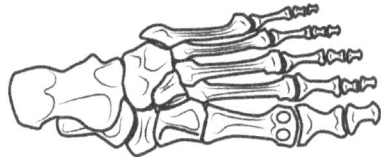

Top View   Bottom View

This different shapes of the tops and bottoms of the tarsal bones also make the surface of the top and bottom of the tarsal joint very different—the top with smooth appearance and the bottom with very jagged appearance.

All this different shapes and sizes of small bones interlocked as a 3D puzzle allow the tarsal joint a very tiny 1-2 mm (about 1/8") of up-and-down range of motion, which is important for absorbing the shock while providing the foot with stability. Because, the foot, the foundation of body, should not fluctuate with a big range of motion—amazingly engineered.

Medial Arch & Lateral Arch

It's important to understand that the foot has high medial arch and low lateral arch.

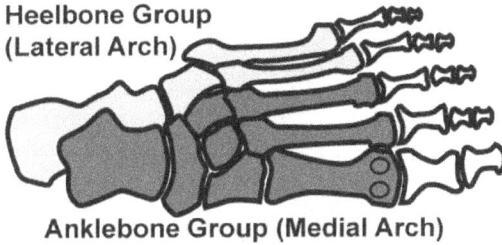

Heelbone Group (Lateral Arch)

Anklebone Group (Medial Arch)

This illustration shows the high medial arch is formed by the anklebone and the bones in front of it. It consists of 8 bones: the anklebone (talus), navicular, 3 cuneiforms, and the 1st, 2nd & 3rd metatarsals. Front of this medial arch connected 3 toes—the big toe, 2nd toe, and 3rd toe—bigger ones among 5 toes.

The low lateral arch is formed by the heel bone and the bones in front of it. It includes 4 bones: the heel bone, cuboid and the 4th & 5th metatarsal bones. This lateral arch sits low—almost to the ground, and its front connects to the 2 toes—the 4th and pinky toes—the smaller ones.

Now we can see the high medial arch is built much stronger having twice as many bones with 3 bigger toes in front of it. On top of that, the plantar muscles beneath the medial arch are about 5 times thicker than beneath the lateral arch.

All this makes perfect sense, since the body weight falls on the anklebone that starts the medial arch. That's why it's crucial keeping our body weight on the medial arch, whether we are standing or walking. Now, let's take a close look at the anklebone and heel bone.

Anklebone

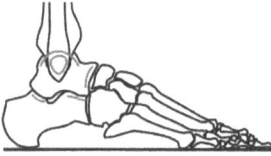 The anklebone has a unique shape with 5 joint areas: 2 joints at the bottom (subtalar joint) sit on the heel bone, on top joint stands the leg bone making the ankle joint, the front joint connects to the navicular, and the joint at the lateral side to the fibular—the slander bone that braces the ankle joint from the outside.

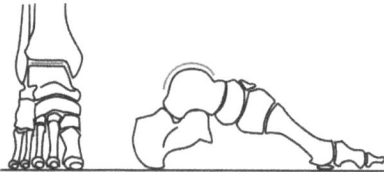 The top of the anklebone from the front view is almost flat with a slight concavity to receive the slight convex bottom of the leg bone (tibia). The side view has a saddle shape, allowing the leg bone to pivot forward and backward.

Now imagine the size of the surface on top of the anklebone where the leg bone stands. It's about 1 square inch. On that tiny space, the leg bone stands with entire body weight and the impact from walking, running, and jumping. This makes the precise alignment of the anklebone absolutely critical.

Heel Bone

Medial View   Lateral View

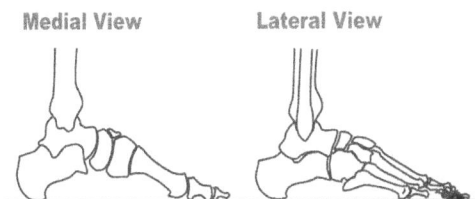

The heel bone stands diagonally with only its back corner touching the ground. This means the actual heel is only the back corner of the heel bone that touches the ground. The Anklebone sits on the front half top of the heel bone—where the bone is suspended diagonally in the air— forms the back part of the arch. The leg stands on the anklebone; so the entire body weight falls on the back part of the arch and then transfers forward through the tarsal joint to the ball of the foot—to make a step.

Front View   Back View

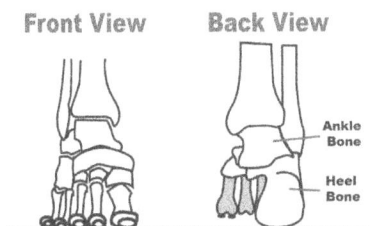

Ankle
Bone

Heel
Bone

This picture shows the leg bone standing on the anklebone. From the back view, notice the empty space right under the medial half of the anklebone. It looks alarming, especially since the bottom of the anklebone slanted medially..!! But thank God, the Engineer of our body machine, filled this space with the thickest foot muscles to cushion the impact from the bodyweight. If this space were filled with bone, it would crack in no time by the impact.

Now, let's look at the soft tissues of the foot: the muscles, ligaments, and tendons.

Soft Tissues of the Foot

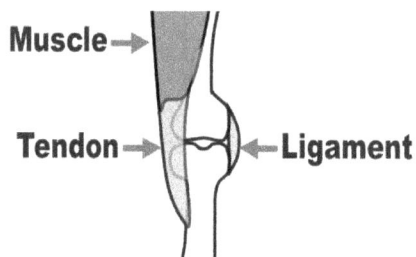

Among the soft tissues, muscles are the most flexible—they move the joints by contracting and relaxing. Tendons connect muscles to bones and have a little flexibility, and ligaments connect bone to bone, and they are the tightest tissues, often embedded firmly into the bones.

The connective tissues are divided into two groups: intrinsic and extrinsic.

Intrinsic Muscles/Ligaments
Intrinsic muscles and ligaments are the tissues that connect the 28 foot bones together to form the foot shape.

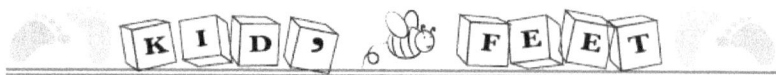

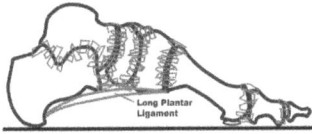

There are over 100 short intrinsic ligaments—hard to count since they are so many of them—interweaving to hold those 28 small bones together. Most of these ligaments are beneath the tarsal joint, and they are called plantar ligaments, tightly connecting those 21 joints with multiple layers of short and medium length ligaments. Some short ligaments connect the toe bones together.

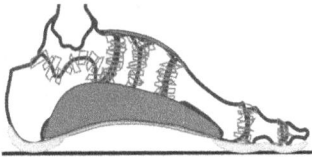

Only a thin layer of muscle covers part of the top of the foot, while most of the foot muscles are beneath those multiple layers of plantar ligaments. These thick muscles are called the "plantar muscles." They are 5 times thicker right under the anklebone, under the medial arch—where the body weight falls—to cushion the impact from the weight.

These plantar muscles work as built-in cushions to absorb the impact that passes down through the tarsal joint. And some fatty tissues are under the heel bone and the ball of the foot to cushion those areas.

Keep in mind: that the heel is only the back part of the heel bone that touches the ground, not the whole rounded area where most people think of as the heel.

The front half of the heel we think as the heel is actually part of the arch.

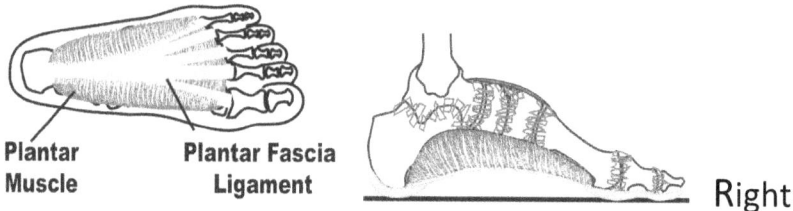

Plantar Muscle   **Plantar Fascia Ligament**

Right beneath the plantar muscles is the plantar fascia ligament that runs from the front bottom of the heel bone and fans out into 5 branches, each attaching to each head of the metatarsal bones in the ball of the foot. This ligament is very tight and can be felt by pressing down along the big toe side of the arch while lifting all the toes up. From both sides of this ligament spread out plethora sheaths of fascia wrapping the plantar muscles and tightly securing them up to the tarsal joint.

Extrinsic Ligaments/Tendons

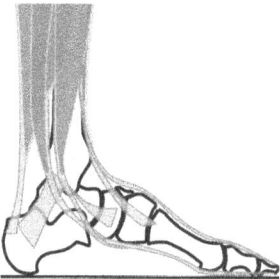

The extrinsic soft tissues of the foot are actually the tendons of the leg muscles originate from the leg bones. And they are the ones move the foot. There are 11 tendons of the leg muscles, all of them passing the ankle joint, and most of them are attached to the bones in the tarsal joint, except the Achilles tendon attach to the back of the heel, and a few long tendons continue forward passing the tarsal joint and attach to the toes to move the toes up and down (toe extensor/flexor).

All of the foot joints and soft tissues function at their best when both anklebones are aligned at the same height with proper orthotics. Even the slightest tilt of the anklebones throws the physical balance.

Tarsal Joint & Orthotics

The tarsal joint is built to handle the impact from our entire body weight—the impact that can reach 3-4 times of our body weight, plus whatever we're carrying. So it can be even more than 10 times of our body weight. Imagine a soldier running with all the combat gears carrying a wounded soldier on their shoulder. Or when kids run, jump, or leap from high places. If there is no proper orthotics, those weight crushes the Tarsal joint misaligning the entire foot bones and the rest of the body that stands on it.

This is why orthotics are essential. But not just any orthotics—the orthotics must align the anklebones at the same height. Only then our feet and the rest of the body can function in alignment without stressing the nerves, joints, muscles, and circulation—all the while minimizing the risk of injury. Because the anklebones connect the feet and the rest of the body, their alignment determines how well everything above and below works together in alignment.

Walking Cycle with Weight

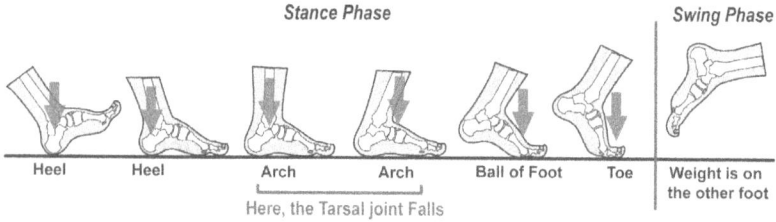

Walking is one of the most basic skills for our daily life. Yet not many people seem to know how to describe it, and, more importantly, how to walk correctly. Walking is simply transferring the body weight from one place to another place on the foot—yet, there is a specific way to do it correctly.

Walking is done by both feet doing 2 different actions at the same time: the stance phase and the swing phase. While one foot stays on the ground carrying the entire body weight (the stance phase), the other foot passes through the air to move the foot forward (the swing phase) before landing on the ground.

Moving a foot through the air is not hard at all because it doesn't carry any weight. But the one on the flat, hard ground carrying the entire body weight is the one doing the hard labor. The feet alternate this hard task with each step, carrying and moving the standing body forward.

Walking requires our body weight pass through the tarsal joint with every step. In this process, the tarsal joint should not fall. But without proper orthotics, the tarsal joint inevitably falls and tilts the anklebone. On tilted anklebones, the body should fall. But our body compensates to keep the body from falling.

This means every step we make, our body is actually falling, and the other foot is catching the falling body as it making a step in front of the falling body. This is how we walk on tilted anklebones—falling and catching, falling and catching—wasting lots of energy.

We just do not realize that's how we walk. This repeated falling-and-catching cycle stresses the entire body by not only wasting energy but all the nerves. However, most people do not realize how this stress affects our body. Only when the anklebones are aligned with proper orthotics, we can get rid of this treacherous cycle and walk correctly without the stress and without falling.

When toddlers are standing, imagine seeing inside of their feet. Their tarsal joints are completely collapsed to the ground under their body weight. When walking, only one foot carries the entire body weight, the fall becomes even more extreme. It's truly remarkable that after few or several falls, toddlers learn to compensate in so many ways, and walk with some wobbles, but without much falling.

Truly, our body is an amazing machine doing all that activities constantly compensating. Sometimes, toddlers say, "Ouch," while walking touching the legs or pointing at the foot, or even crying at night holding their feet. Yes, they are walking with their entire foot ligaments and tendons twisting and pulling with each step all day. If they are born to have tight muscles, the ligaments that have been twisting all day can be inflamed and cause pain even at that early age. Children born with flexible muscles would not have pain from inflammation, but they will suffer more joint damage down the road.

Many parents worry when their children having flat feet or pain. Some take their children to healthcare professionals and are told that they will "grow out of it," while others try some insoles. But their feet only grow out of alignment, unless they use the orthotics that aligning their anklebones at the same height, the feet and major joint problems would not be properly treated or healed. Because the arch at the bottom of our foot was meant to be supported.

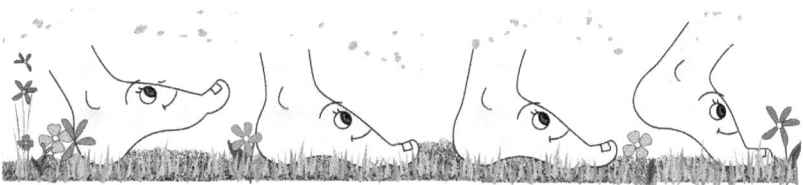

Long, long ago, in the Garden of Eden, people walked barefoot on soft soil. That soft soil supported the arch perfectly.

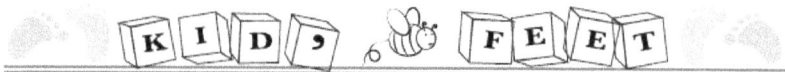

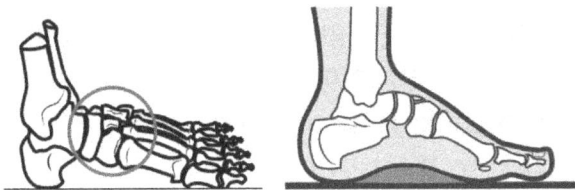

That's why the tarsal joint didn't fall. So the feet were happy— walking, running, and jumping around with balance and comfort. When our feet are happy, our body standing on them is happy too.

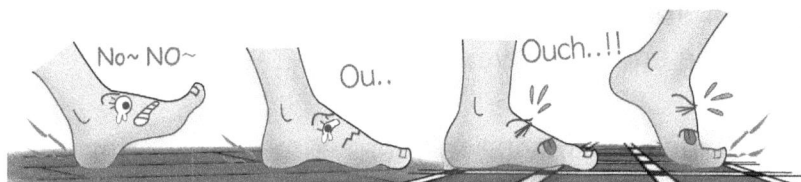

But now, with industrialization, the ground we walk has become literally flat and hard—wood, concrete, and even tile or marble floors—with no means of supporting the tarsal joint—and children live on them.

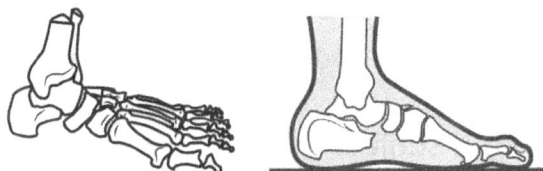

On these flat, hard floors, the tarsal joint inevitably falls, and the feet end up walking, running, or jumping with all the foot bones out of alignment, so the rest of the body.

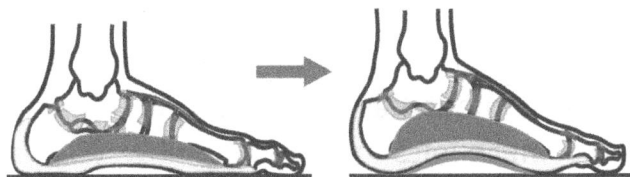

For the foot to function in alignment, all we need to do is

using proper orthotics that aligning both anklebones at the same height. Then our feet will be happy again—being able to walk, run, and jump around with balance and comfort, so the rest of the body.

Purpose of Alignment

We all know how critical it is for a machine to move with proper alignment for the machine to perform well and last long. Then what exactly does alignment provide for the machine to run smoothly and function well wile enduring over time?

Many people having a hard time answering this question, often responding with something like, "Because it is . . . aligned." or "It's aligned, that is why . . ." not really answering the question.

The answer is simple: **"Even Weight Distribution."** Alignment = Even Weight Distribution = Minimal Deterioration = Optimal Functionality for a long time.

Every object on earth is subject to gravity, that is why every joint—whether it's a machine or a human body—wears down over time under weight or pressure, even with proper alignment. Without the alignment, deterioration happens faster and more severely—due to uneven weight distribution. Especially, areas that deal with heavy weight or pressure, the alignment has to be very precise. For example, auto mechanics understand how a small piece of lead on the wheels affects the alignment and performance of the entire vehicle.

Just like a wheel, the anklebone carries our entire body weight. The area on top of the anklebone where the leg bone stands with the entire body weight is about one square inch, on fully grown anklebone, which is still extremely small when you consider how much weight falls on it. That is why the anklebone alignment demands extremely precise alignment.

In fact, inch for inch, our anklebone can withstand more weight than the tires of average vehicles that weigh about 4,000 pounds.

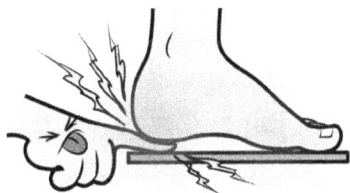 Because the bottom of the foot is designed incredibly for tremendous weight-bearing, people do not realize how much weight falls at the bottom of the foot. (Curious? Put a finger under someone else's heel. This will hurt but instantly let you know.) Imagine when we jump around, sometimes carrying all kinds of heavy stuffs too.

Think of ballet dancers swirling on the ball of the foot, leaping and landing on a single foot, and even standing on their toes—with their entire body weight and impact that can be several hundred pounds. This damages the foot in so many ways. Even though they cannot use orthotics while dancing or any activity, right after the activity, they should use the orthotic for their feet to rest and heal with proper alignment.

Even with proper orthotics, our body generates a lot of pressure between the orthotics and the bottom of the foot. That is why even a tiny grain of sand or a small lint from a sock inside of the shoes feel irritating and has to be removed. Because of this tightness, even one post card (less than a 1/2 mm) thickness between orthotics and the foot sole disrupts even weight distribution and breaks the balance. Then the body will fail the Anklebone Alignment Test. It's like a slight invisible dent on a eyeglass lens that distorts the vision.

Also, we can think of not using orthotics as kind of torturing the foot in the opposite way of Chinese binding foot that bends the tarsal joint upward to put them in extremely tight shoes. Without the orthotics, we are bending the tarsal joint downward with our entire body weight against flat surfaces with each step—demanding bigger shoe size.

Odd-Shaped Body Joints

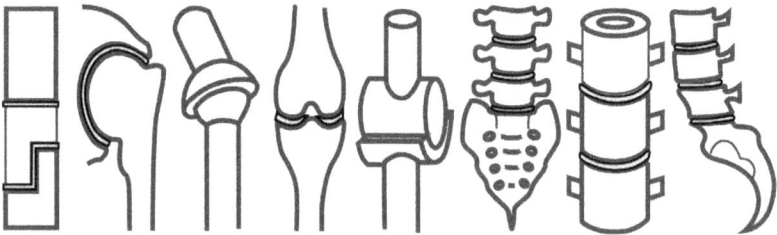

Our body joints are oddly shaped with all different range of motion. This makes it difficult to say if any given angle of a joint is from within its normal range of motion or from out of alignment. However, we can tell the difference between the two with strength test and use of the range of motion. If the angle of a joint is from within its range of motion, the body should be able to utilize its full strength and its full range of motion. But even a slightest angle of the joint is from out of alignment, the body cannot utilize its full strength and its full range of motion—the simple logic that helped me to developed Anklebone Alignment Test.

Ironically, we—the most intelligent being on earth—understand that every machine should be aligned before put into operation, do not apply that same concept to our own body machine, and, furthermore, some people even think having one leg shorter than the other—proof of our body moving out of alignment—as normal..!

Why the alignment matters. First of all, the alignment of our body should be checked in a standing posture, not while laying down. Because that is when our body weight affects the joints.

If the alignment is done on a lying down posture on a flat surface like puzzle pieces, when our body stands up on the feet, the tarsal joint falls instantly—throwing the body out of alignment.

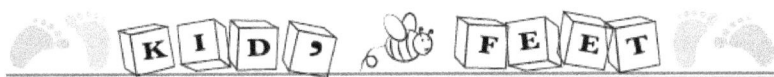

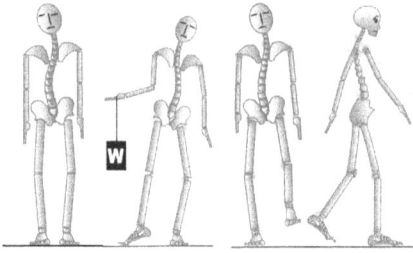

When you think about, a body standing out of alignment cannot develop its full strength. It's like its full strength locked away in every misaligned joint. On top of that, the limited strength we've developed—with the body that is out of alignment—we cannot use that strength fully either. Because this body has to compensate constantly. This compensation limits the range of motion while wasting energy also, and make the body vulnerable to injuries. Another thing is this misaligned body keeps damaging the foot and major joints.

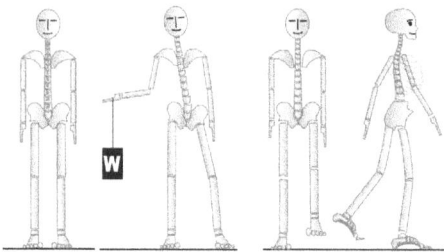

In contrast, aligned body can develop its full strength and doesn't need to compensate. So this body can use its full strength and full range of motion, and reduces the risk of injury, such as sprains, strains, and overuse problems, and the body can perform at its best with good posture.

Another benefit is when the body gets jerked around in any accident, the body in alignment gets less damage than the body out of alignment.

It's like without proper orthotics, our body getting slapped twice and thrice.

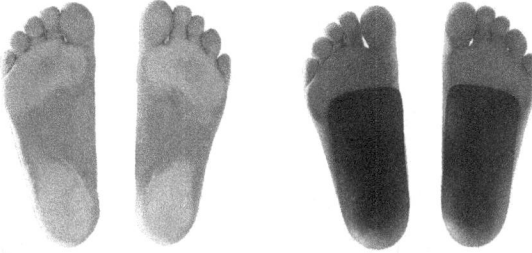

The photo on the left shows the feet bottoms standing on a clear plastic. We can see the arch area (designed to carry 75% of the weight) not carrying the weight, instead, the heel and the ball of the foot handling the most body weight—the reason socks having holes in those areas.

This concentrated pressure squeezes blood out from these areas, turning them white. This hinders the overall circulation since the blood vessels are all interconnected. The photo on the right shows the feet with proper orthotics that align the anklebones. This spreads the body weight evenly at the bottom of the foot including the arch area, and allows the blood to circulate.

Walking barefoot on streets scattered with broken glasses damages our body from outside, mostly the skin of the feet. But walking on flat, hard floors damages our body from inside—the joints, ligaments, tendons, and nerves—leading to more serious damages.

Fallen tarsal joint pulls and twists the entire ligaments and tendons in and around the foot. Then the toes grab the ground. This toe grabbing can develop into hammertoes down the road. Also, both tarsal joints usually fall in different ways making every human body structure asymmetrical.

The orthotics that align the anklebones can release all the connective tissues (ligaments, tendons, and muscles) to their proper places. Then the entire skeletomuscular system can grow and move with alignment without pulling, twisting, and pinching.

(While working at Disney my jaw dropped when my chiropractor showed me the x-ray film of my spine with severe scoliosis. It looked almost like a question mark—without the dot. And my right leg was about an inch shorter than my left leg. However, I had never felt I was limping and my spine being out of alignment. I always thought I had a good posture. After I align my anklebones with orthotics for about a couple years, a chiropractor checked my spine at a health fair and said he hasn't seen anybody with such a straight spine like mine. I knew my orthotics aligned my anklebones; thus, my leg length became the same, systematically aligning my hip bones; and on aligned hips, my spine started to change its course and straightened out by itself.)

When your kids start venturing out to stand and walk at around the age of 1, supporting your kid's arch with little cookie shaped orthotics would do its job. If it's done correctly, you can see them walking steadier without much staggering or falling.

☆Think about This

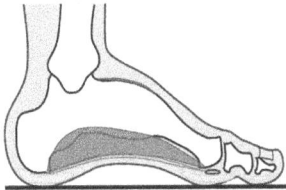 If the arch is made with one big bone without any joint, our major joints can keep its alignment, but still the foot needs orthotics to carry the body weight throughout the bottom of the foot, including the arch part.

Notes

Chapter 2

Kid's Foot & the Arch

How Kid's Foot Grows

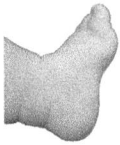

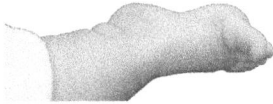

If you look at every newborn baby's feet, you can see the arch at the bottom of their feet—even though their foot bones are not yet complete in shape and number.

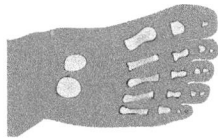

This X-ray drawing of newborn baby foot shows only 2 bones (the heel bone and the anklebone) of the 7 tarsal bones, but all the 5 metatarsal bones and toe bones are there.

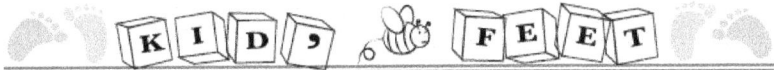

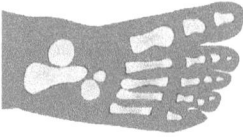

At around ages of 1-2 years old, a few more tarsal bones begin to appear.

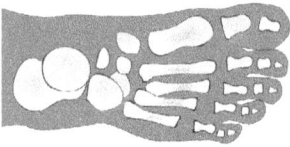

By around ages of 3-4 years old, all the foot bones are present.

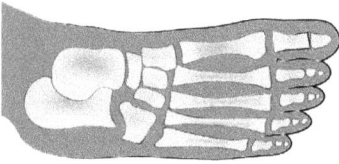

At around ages of 5-7, the gaps between the joints close in as the bones start taking on their unique shapes.

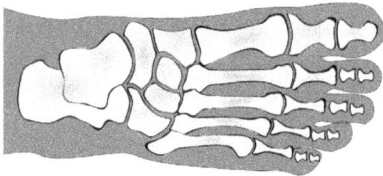

By ages of 8-10, most foot bones seem to take their unique shapes, and they continue growing in sizes until they reach their gene's intended full size at around ages of 15-16.

However, the navicular bone—in front of the anklebone—calcifies last. This is why proper orthotics are so important during childhood. They help all the developing bones to grow in alignment, especially, the navicular that needs space to grow and calcify without being squeezed by the surrounding bones that have already calcified.

Once our feet reach their full size around age 16, that's it. They don't grow anymore. If you think their feet keep growing after their 16th birthday, that is because their tarsal joint—the arch—keeps falling with each step making their arch longer and wider—making the foot longer and wider—not from growing.

The Arch & Orthotics

The arch is constructed with tarsal joint and numerous soft tissues, the ligaments and thick muscles under it for cushioning for weight bearing. To utilize this arch properly for its function, proper orthotics are essential.

Here are some x-ray drawings of children's foot making a step without and with orthotics.

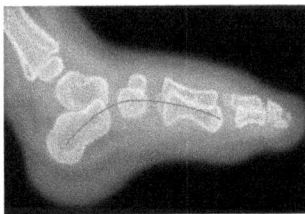

This x-ray illustration shows a toddler's tarsal joint nicely arranged forming the arch, before making a step.

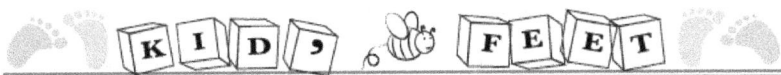

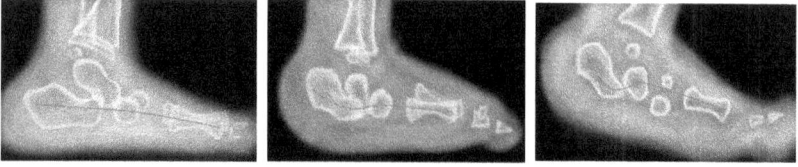

These illustrations show when toddlers make a step on a flat floor, their still-developing tarsal joint with super-flexible ligaments falls completely flattening the arch—the flat foot. This puts all the foot bones out of alignment.

Basically, the flat foot is "a foot with complete-fallen-tarsal joint," or "a complete-fallen-arched foot," which is a deformed foot—even though it may still look cute from outside.

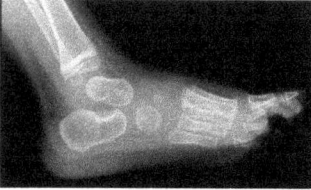

Another x-ray image of before making a step shows the tarsal joint nicely arranged forming the arch.

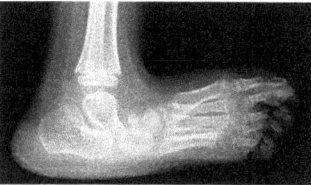

But when the foot makes a step, the tarsal joint collapses completely, putting all the foot bones out of alignment—the arch completely collapsed. Imagine all the foot ligaments and tendons overstretching and twisting to wrong directions.

This happens to children's tarsal joint with each step they make.

Now, we understand why the orthotics are essential device for our foot.

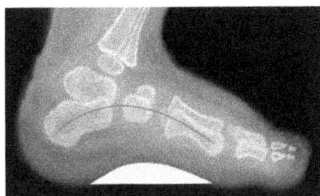

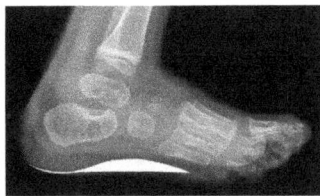

When making a step with orthotics under the arch, the tarsal joint cannot fall—so keeps its alignment in an arch shape, so the foot bones can grow in alignment.

Tarsal Joint & Screws

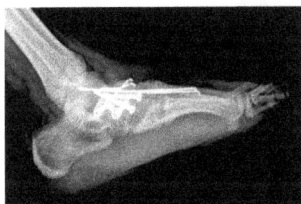

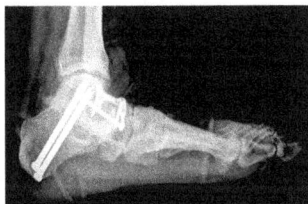

Please, the tarsal joint and screws do not go together. The screws can never, ever, forever align the anklebones. Can't you see the stress the tarsal joint is getting from the screws with each step as our body weight falls on it? Without proper orthotics, the impact on the tarsal joint eventually loosens its grip and starts fluctuating, and the screws can even pop out of the skin.

Even if the screws have to be installed for some reason—though I cannot imagine why, since orthotics and proper binding can stabilize even a damaged tarsal joint—first we need to use proper orthotics and install the screws. In that way the screws can be installed properly in alignment, and those screws won't pop out either.

Notes

Chapter 3

Growing on Tilted Anklebones

In This Chapter
- Scoliosis
- Rickets
- Kids Major Joint Pain
- Normal Damage & Extra Damage
- Just for a Thought

When toddlers are ready to venture out from their crawling life to walking life, they already developed an excellent sense of physical balance. So when their tarsal joints fall as they stand on flat floors, they instantly sense something is wrong—they cannot balance their bodies..!! And they cannot communicate that verbally as well. All they can do is wishing for their parents recognize their ordeal by their awkward standing with grabbing toes or falling.

One fortunate thing is that no pain yet, because all their soft tissues—the ligaments and tendons—are super flexible and ample space between the joints won't let the joints knocking each other to cause pain.

But their parents—delighted to see their toddlers finally standing—clapping their hands and laughing at how cute they look: their awkward standing, wobbly walking, even falling. They totally oblivious to the struggle their kids are going through.

Wouldn't toddlers be confused? They are going through hard time, yet, their parents are celebrating. What an irony and harsh reality from the start..!!

However, they have to survive. This situation forces them to compensate in many ways—so they won't fall. I wonder if this early frustration prompts them to yell "No" or something not kind... Oh dear, did I go too far..?

Whenever there is a danger of falling, our body instinctively compensates.

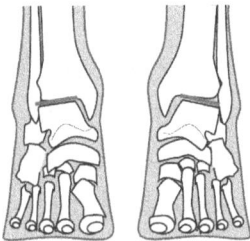

 On tilted anklebones, our body is consistently in danger of falling. Then our brain makes our body to compensate at each weight-bearing joints to keep our body from falling. That is how our body stands in a zigzag manner. I call this zigzag standing, "the primary compensatory behavior," which we cannot undo unless we align our tilted anklebone to the same height with proper orthotics.

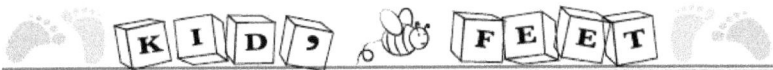

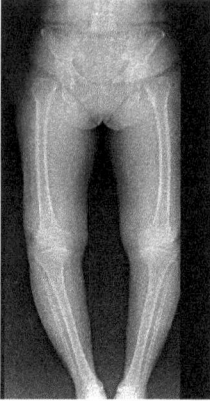

This teenager's x-ray shows bowlegs with damages (the white spots indicate stress or damage) in the inner side of the knee joint. Because bowlegs compress the inner side of the joint.

Why does this child have bowlegs? Look at the anklebones at the bottom. Both anklebones tilted laterally (outward) with different angles and heights, because both tarsal joints' usual fall with different degrees and angles. This weakens the ankle joint and can easily sprain the joint. The left anklebone tilted outward more than the right, while the right anklebone is lower than the left. This means the left tarsal joint fell more to the outside, while the right tarsal joint fell more forward.

Because the tarsal joint is located in front of anklebone, when it falls, the anklebone always tilts forward and goes off sideways as well. That is why, in most cases, the anklebones tilt diagonally, misaligning the rest of the body structure diagonally as well—the leg bones, hip bones, and the spine, and even the head.

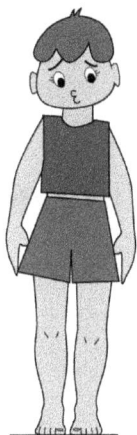

Tell your kids to stand straight and observe their posture closely. If your eyes are trained, you can see a lot.

Start checking the leg-length difference by pressing down at both tops of the hip bones (iliac crests) with your fingertips. And see which side is lower. Most children, even adults, have one leg shorter than the other, meaning their hip bones are tilted. You can also check different heights in their kneecaps by pressing up against the bottom of the kneecaps with the index fingers (or short sticks). You can see one kneecap is slightly lower than the other.

On tilted hip bones, the spine can only stand with some degree of scoliosis. Although this twisted spine may not be obvious from outside, the tilted shoulder line and one shoulder blade higher than the other prove the scoliosis. Look closely at the face: the mouthline, nose, eyes, and ears are all slightly tilted to one side. Also, when they raise their head, you might be able to see their one side of the jaw is lower than the other side.

Finally, observe their feet. Usually, one foot is slightly wider than the other.

All this asymmetry starts from the bottom as both tarsal joints falling differently, because most of us use one side foot predominantly.

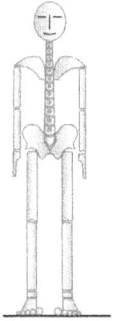 On aligned anklebones, the spine should look straight from the front view.

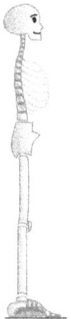 However, from the side, the spine has its nice natural curve from the bottom. The bottom part (Lumbar), where the digestive system (fuel tank) located, curves forward to give more room for the stomach and intestines to move easily to digest and make our body to bend at the waist for many tasks. The meddle part (Thoracic) curves backward with the rib cage in front to give a nice round space to store the critical parts—the heart (engine), the lungs

(exhaust system), and livers (lubricant system). The upper part (cervical), the neck, curves forward to put the head that needs to look forward most of time. Incredible design..!

I think the number of the vertebra starting from the top like L1, L2... confuses people to think the alignment our entire body structure starts from the top, which doesn't make sense at all. If the number starts from bottom—just like the floors of buildings— might help people to understand our body alignment also starts at the bottom.

Scoliosis

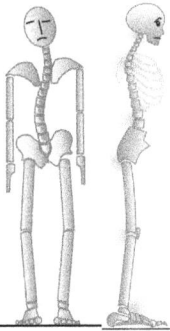

The tendency of the tarsal joint falling diagonally misaligns the entire body structure diagonally. This makes our body stands in a zigzag manner from the front and side views, even the spine. That is why the spine goes out of alignment from the front and side views.

As mentioned earlier, body alignment should be checked in a standing posture, when the major joints are carrying the body weight—not while lying down.

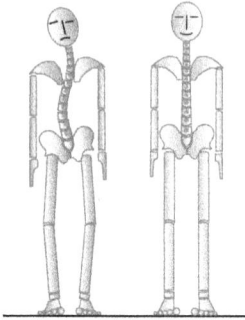

On the tilted anklebone, it's impossible for the leg to stand straight unless you compensate at the ankle joint 100%, which will make very weak ankle. Also, both tarsal joints falling differently make one leg shorter than the other. With one leg shorter than the other, one cannot avoid limping. Believe it or not, most, if not all, people are limping to some degree. Yes, including you.

Another consequence of the fallen tarsal joints is that your kid's overall height becomes shorter than their actual height; because a body standing in a zigzag manner is shorter than the one standing in alignment.

Rickets

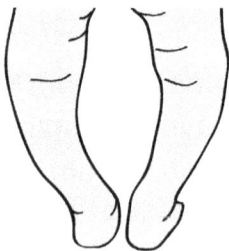

The common cause of rickets is known for the lack of vitamin D or calcium. However, the legs standing on the laterally tilted anklebones (supination) can grow into a bow shape. That is why most, if not all, x-ray images of the kids with this

Rickets disease have tilted anklebones. The growing out of alignment cannot grow strong and the ligaments and tendons cannot develop its strength fully either. Also, walking with the tilted anklebones stresses the whole central nerve system and consumes more energy than walking with aligned anklebones.

The orthotics can surely improve the condition of Rickets with other vitamin D and calcium treatment. If some rickets could have developed from the fallen tarsal joint, just aligning the anklebones with proper orthotics surely prevent and improve the condition.

Kids Major Joint Pain

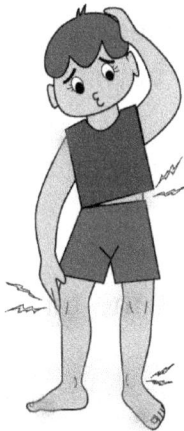

Some kids, as early as 4 or 5 years old, already complain about pains on their feet, and even on the major joints such as ankles, knees, back, or neck. Most people think these pains as growing pain. But, most likely, they are from moving their body without the alignment due to their tilted anklebones. (There was an article, "Orthotics can help Kids'

Growing Pains," by the Pedorthic Association of Canada [www.pedorthic.ca] in February 2012 stating that the orthotics helped growing pain.)

When I was teaching 4 year old kids in Sunday school, one boy walked straight towards me as he was entering the classroom and tugged gently at the corner of my sweater and telling me a story with a serious facial expression:

"Teacher, teacher, my knees hurt... So I told my mom that my knees hurt. But my mom told me that my knees don't hurt. But teacher, my knees REALLY hurt..."

This is exactly what the boy had said word for word emphasizing at the word "REALLY." It sounded like his mom not believing what he said was true bewildered him. I saw a little disappointment in this boy's little eyes that caused by his own parents not believing him when he said what was true.

It's so important to educate people about the tarsal joint in need of orthotics to align the anklebones to prevent the feet and major joint problems—starting from toddlers. Some children get physical therapy, but the feet and major joint problems would not be fixed until they align their tilted anklebones.

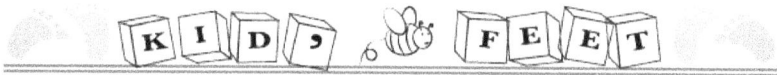

KIDS FEET

Normal Damage & Extra Damage

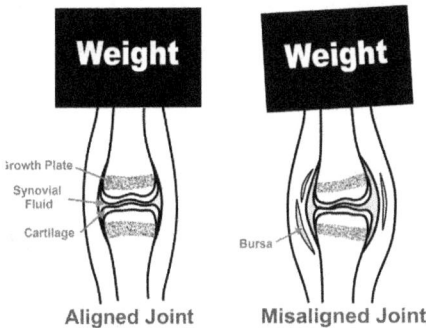

Growth Plate

Synovial Fluid

Cartilage

Weight

Weight

Bursa

Aligned Joint

Misaligned Joint

Weight-bearing joints deteriorates even with alignment. Let's call this natural deterioration "normal damage." Thankfully, our body machine Manufacturer made our body to lie down at night, for about 8 hours—not bearing any weight. During this time, the blood, our body's amazing healing agent, can easily reach into the relaxed joints more efficiently, delivering good things in and bad things out with each breath and revitalizes the normal damage. So technically, all of the normal damage that happens during the daytime should be fully recovered while sleeping. As a result, the next day, the body machine should be all refreshed and ready to function fully well again.

But on the tilted anklebones, the body moving out of alignment, causes "extra damage" to the weight-bearing joints. Then the 8 hour sleep would not be enough to heal the normal and the extra damage fully, even though the healing system works harder all night. So next morning, the body wakes up with a bit of residue of unhealed damage on every weight-

43

bearing joint. As time passes by, the portion of unhealed damage gets bigger and bigger, and, eventually, makes our body to function noticeably difficult.

Yet, most of us aren't aware of this accumulating residual damage, until pain suddenly starts one day, and not being able to do some activities as they used to. Also, this damage demands our body to spend more time sitting and lying down—to give more time to heal the damage.

☆ Just for a thought

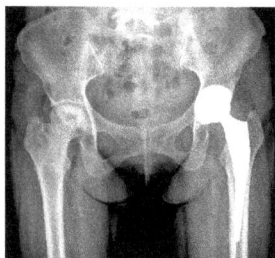

This is not a kid's hip x-ray. It's an adult's hip x-ray after a hip replacement surgery with the replaced hip joint higher than the other side. This obviously tilts the hip bones. When replacing any major joint, shouldn't making both leg lengths the same be one of the goals of the surgery? So that this person can walk without limping.

We can see most hip x-ray images on the Internet are in a tilted position with or without the hip replacement surgery.

Notes

Chapter 4

Fallen Tarsal Joint & Foot Deformities

In This Chapter
- Flat Foot
- Curled Toes
- Bunion
- Protrusion of 5th Metatarsal Root
- splay Foot
- Callus
- Pigeon Toes
- Tip Toeing
- They will Never Grow Out of It

Let's talk about how toddlers' feet begin to deform from their very first step as their tarsal joints fall. Even though their tarsal joint completely collapses to the ground, due to their super-flexible-ligaments, most kids don't feel pain; except a few (who are born to have real tight muscles) might cry out at night holding their feet due to inflamed plantar ligaments because their tarsal joint falling all day.

Most foot deformities can be prevented—and even be improved by using proper orthotics.

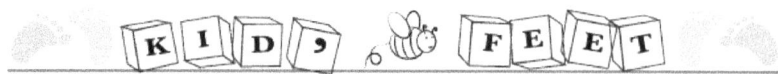

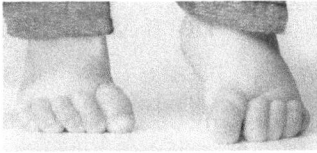

Can you see these baby feet...

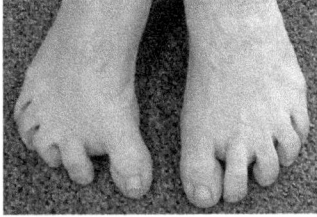

transforming to these feet...?

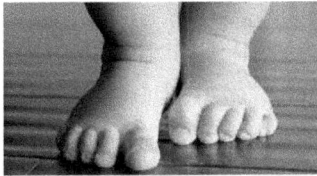

And these feet...

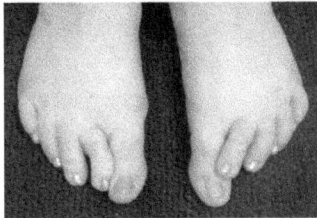

to these...?

Flat Foot

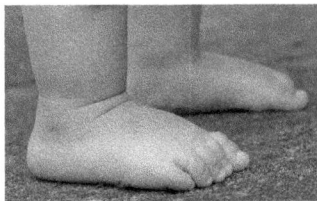

This toddler's feet may still look cute with complete fallen tarsal joint—the flat feet—which are already deformed feet. The grabbing toes are the child's attempt to keep the tarsal joint from farther falling. Also, they try to help the ball of the foot by lifting a portion of the weight from it.

As mentioned earlier, no one is ever born with flat feet—unless it's a birth defect. Even in a rare case of a baby born with flat feet as a birth defect, orthotics should be used alongside with any needed medical treatment—for their foot bones to grow in alignment with an arch at the bottom.

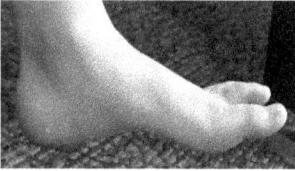

This is a 5-year-old boy's foot before making a step. The arch is there at the bottom.

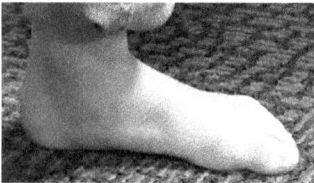

Now, the foot makes a step and the arch collapses quite a bit (this boy has tight muscles, otherwise the arch would disappear completely). This pulls and squeezes all the soft tissues (ligaments, tendons, nerves, etc.) in the foot to wrong directions and stresses them.

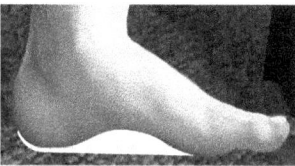

With proper orthotics, his foot should look more like this.

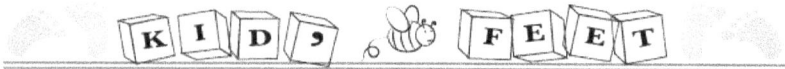

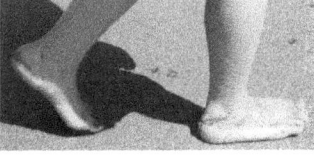

This image shows a 7-year-old boy, born with flexible muscles, walking on a beach. You can see the arch in his left foot before making a step—not carrying any weight yet.

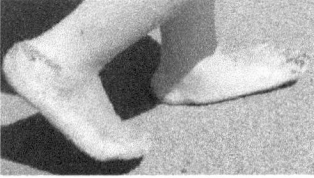

Now, the left foot makes a step carrying his entire body weight—as the other foot is lifted from the ground—the arch completely collapses and becomes a flat foot. Can you imagine all the foot bones now being out of alignment—including the anklebone, and so his entire body structure?

This has been happening with every step since he was a toddler. But he doesn't feel any pain or discomfort yet . . . until when? Who knows . . . He just needs the orthotics as soon as possible for his feet and his body structure to grow in alignment and prevent all the problems of the tilted anklebones down the road.

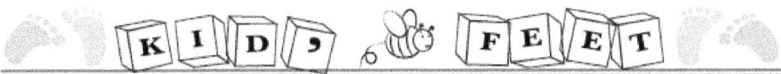

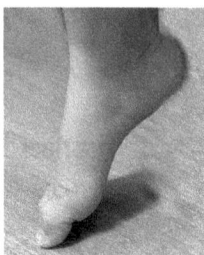

This 3 year old kid's foot with a nice arch—not carrying body weight.

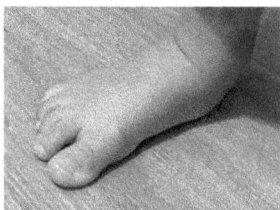

After making a step, the arch disappears.

Curled Toes

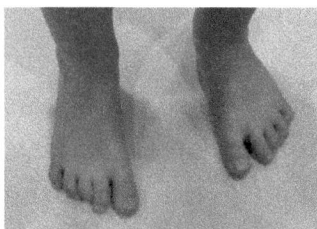

This is 4 years old kid's feet with curled toes. Toes are attached to the front of the metatarsal bones that are part of the tarsal joint.

When the tarsal joint falls, those 5 metatarsal bones fall while twisting in different directions. Then the toes attached to the metatarsal heads twist alongside to all different directions and angles while grabbing the ground. This toe grabbing can develop into hammertoes down the road.

And the left foot is wider than the right indicates both tarsal joints falling differently, deforming both feet differently.

Bunion

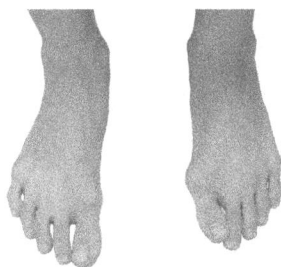

It's hard to believe these are the feet of an 8-year-old girl—with bunions and tailor bunions (a bump at the pinky toe side). These bunions and tailor bunions develop as the tarsal joints fall and rise with each step inside narrow-toe-box-shoes.

Every step the foot makes, the tarsal joint falls, elongating and widening the arch. Then both sides of the ball of the foot rub against the shoe wall moving forward, and as the foot lifted from the ground, the arch recoils—causing them rubbing backward.

Imagine this back-and-forth rubbing happens 2500-5000 times a day per foot (based on the average 5,000-10,000 steps a day). This frequent friction can develop bunion and tailer bunion at that early age—even deforming the shoe shape.

Also, callus can build up on top of the bunion as it rubs the top of the shoe wall. Or, when people walk around with bare feet in shoes with vinyl shoe wall, the skin on the side of the ball of the foot can stick to the vinyl while the metatarsal head rubbing back and forth inside the skin. This can cause the affected skin to become thin and red.

Protrusion of 5th Metatarsal Root

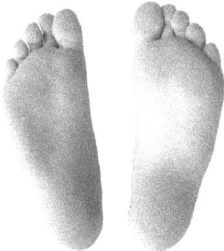

The feet bottoms of 9 year old kid with a little bump at the lateral arch. Even without carrying any weight, the foot bones are all out of alignment. The bumps would become worse when standing. This happens when the tarsal joint falls mostly toward the outside, flattening the wide root of the 5th metatarsal bone against the floor.

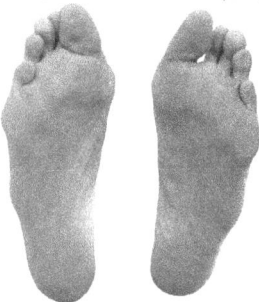

60 years later, above 9 year old foot bottoms can become like these feet bottoms of a 69 year old.

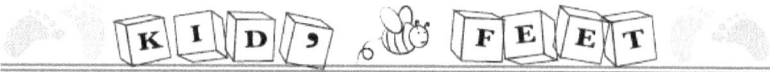

Splay Foot

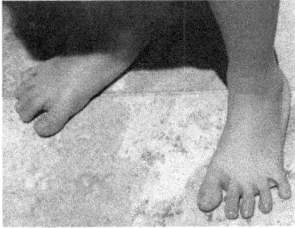

This 4-year-old kid standing on marble floor with bare feet. The arch fell flat to the floor, and toes are all splayed out indicating the kid born with flexible muscles. These spread-out toes may have happened in an attempt to cover more ground to stabilize the foot. Also, notice the fatty skin under the left heel is squished out against the flat floor.

Callus

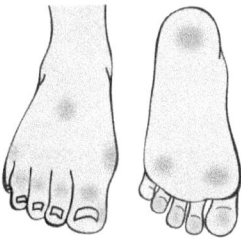

Calluses can build up all over the foot by uneven weight and friction against all around the inside the shoes. Without proper orthotics, the weight only goes to the heel, ball of the foot, and toes, causing callus to build up on those areas. And as the tarsal joint falls and rises with each step, the callus can develop on top of the foot and tops of the grabbing toes by the friction against the shoe ceiling.

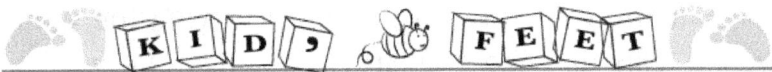

Pigeon Toes

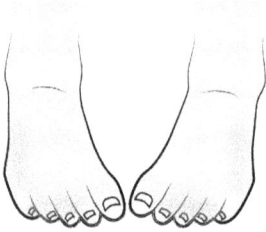

In an attempt to prevent the high medial arch (big toe side) from falling, some kids instinctively turn the feet medially. This puts the most body weight to the lateral arch, which is much lower and weaker, causing the complete collapse of the lateral arch. This is known as pigeon toeing or in-toeing. When this gets severe, both feet turn medially to the point of putting the side of the foot almost to the front; this pigeon toeing twists the ankle joints, thus, knee joints and hip joint. In extreme cases, it can even dislocate the hip joint.

Tip Toeing

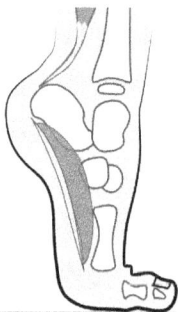

Some kids instinctively walk on their ball of the foot lifting the heel. This makes the tarsal joint stack on top of each other, so the joint wouldn't fall. But the ball of the foot alone carrying the entire weight can damage the area; causing severe callus build up, and if the circulation cuts off really bad, even open ulcers can happen.

Also, this tip toeing shortens the Achilles tendon while overstretching the ligaments and tendons in front of the ankle joint. So when they try to correct their walking, it would be difficult, especially, due to the shortened Achilles tendon.

They wil Never Grow Out of It

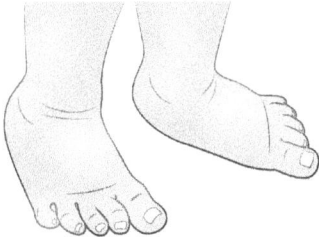

Kids having flat feet and curled toes are the result of the fallen tarsal joints. They will not grow out of them. Yet, most healthcare providers do not think it's necessary for toddlers to use orthotics. So aligning kids' tilted anklebones falls into your hands. Get them orthotics if you want your children's body to grow in alignment from the feet up.

Toddler's feet grow pretty fast, so the size of orthotics should be changed when their shoe size changes. Even a little bit of support is better than nothing, because they keep the tarsal joint from complete collapsing.

Notes

Chapter 5

Fallen Tarsal Joint & Foot Pain

Out of aligned joints cause pain—sooner or later.

Why Fallen Tarsal Joint Itself Has No Pain

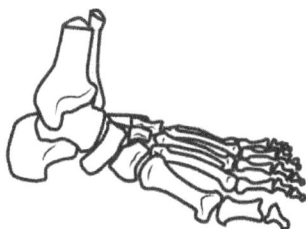

Now we know when the tarsal joint falls, the entire foot bones go out of alignment, including the anklebone, and causes foot pain. However, the tarsal joint itself, on top of the foot, rarely has pain. Because while falling, tarsal joint compensates with 21 Joints in all different directions—to alleviate pain.

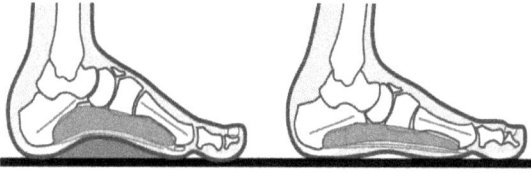

Also, when tarsal joint falls, the space between the joints spread out making the foot flatter and wider. This keeps the joints from knocking each other, unless someone wears very tight shoes.

Consequently, most pain caused by the fallen tarsal joint happens at the bottom of the foot and in the major joints above the anklebones. Now, let's go over the foot pain.

Heel Pain

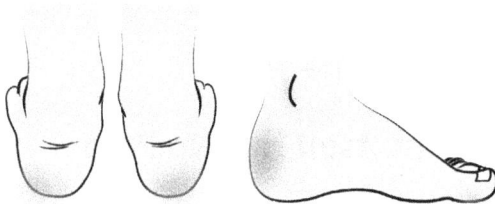

When the tarsal joint falls, the heel bone rotates backward while shifting out of alignment. This pulls and twists all the ligaments and tendons around the heel bone, which can cause pain all around the heel; pain at the back of the heel caused by pulling and twisting of the Achilles tendon; pain at the side can happen by pulling the ligaments and tendons on both sides of the heel bone. Also, the heel area handling a lot more weight with the heel bone out of alignment can cause pain too.

Ball of the Foot Pain

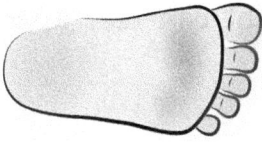

The ball of the foot carrying a lot more weight than it's designed for with all the metatarsal bones out of alignment can damage the ball of the foot and cause pain there. This symptom is known as "Metatarsalgia,"

Stubbed Toe

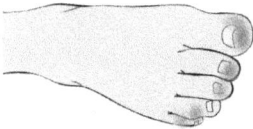

These stubbed toe injuries can happen when tarsal joint falls inside shoes without enough toe box space for the elongated foot to stretch forward. As a result, the toes slamming against the front of the shoe inside with each step. Over time, this repeated slamming can bruise the tips of the toes

Plantar Fasciitis

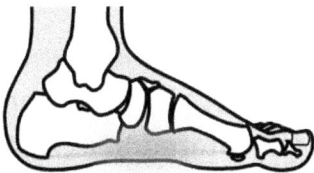

Plantar fasciitis is an inflammation of the plantar fascia ligament—the longest ligament that runs from the front bottom of the heel bone to the back of the metatarsal heads.

When tarsal joint falls, the arch elongates, over-stretching the plantar fascia ligament. When it falls severely, the tissues of this ligament can tear apart and can causes pain.

Although plantar fasciitis usually affects adults, children born with tight muscles can have pain from this plantar fasciitis. Even toddlers cry out at night holding their feet. These kids may have been born to have tight muscles. So during the day while walking on flat, hard floors, this ligament can be overstretched and become inflamed at night and cause pain.

Children complaining pain after playing any activities that involve running or jumping, most of them would be from fallen tarsal joint. Once you get them proper orthotics, they can enjoy those activities without the foot and major joint pain.

Heel Spur

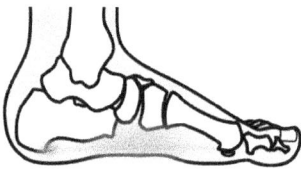

In some cases, as the plantar fascia ligament overstretches, it can tear apart from the front edge of the heel bone that rotated backward and facing the floor, and carrying the weight. Think about the situation. The front edge of the heel bone—which should be facing forward, so shouldn't carry any body weight—carrying the body weight while the ligament attached there over-stretched. Doesn't it sound so ouch? Yet, amazingly, the pain doesn't always start right away.

As time passes by, uric acid that has been gathered at the bottom of the foot—due to poor circulation there—get into the torn apart area and absorb calcium from the bone or the ligament. Over time, it gradually forms into a thorn shape bone growth at the front of the heel bone, which known as "heel spur." Walking with a heel spur can be very painful. We can see this heel spur as the second stage of plantar fasciitis.

Some people get cortisone shots for both the plantar fasciitis and heel spur conditions. But cortisone can make living tissues brittle—almost glass-like—and can permanently damage their ability to heal. Others undergo plantar release surgery, which partially cut the plantar fascia ligament to prevent the overstretching. Although this procedure can relieve pain rather quickly, it would be better to take pain killer. Because releasing the ligament by cutting allows the tarsal joint to fall more easily, and so our body moves with worse alignment—boosting the major joints deterioration worse.

Surprisingly, despite the severe pain caused by plantar fasciitis and heel spur, using proper orthotics often relieves the pain almost immediately. It's like a pain from a misaligned joint relieves instantly when the joint is put back to its alignment.

Most people should assume that they have some degree of inflammation in this plantar fascia ligament. They just don't realize it until pain suddenly starts, usually, in the morning, the moment they take the first step out of bed, or when standing up after sitting for a while.

There is a reason why the foot pain starts after it seemed to have plenty of rest. It's because, while sitting or lying down, tarsal joint won't fall—so the ligament doesn't overstretch. During that time, the connective tissues start repairing the damaged ligament. But when we stand up again, the tarsal joint falls again, tearing apart the partially healed ligament; That tearing is what triggers the "Ouch!" pain. As we continue walking, the pain may subside as the tearing process is over.

As this tearing-and-healing cycle repeats every day, the inflammation worsens, and walking can become very difficult because of severe pain. Also, this tearing-and-healing cycle can cause scar tissue build-ups along the ligament and can feel like bumpy knots in the arch.

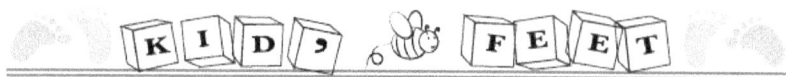

KID' FEET

Achilles Tendonitis

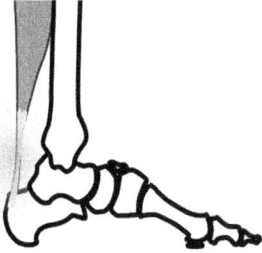

As the tarsal joint falls throughout the day, the heel bone keeps tilting or twisting with every step, torquing the Achilles tendon; this can eventually inflame the tendon and cause pain.

Kohler's Disease

Kohler's disease happens when the navicular bone is unable to develop normally. Let's see how this happens.

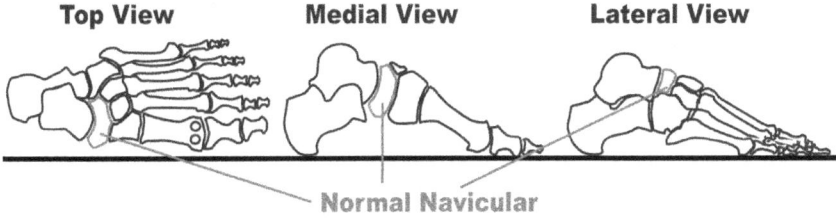

Top View   **Medial View**   **Lateral View**

Normal Navicular

The navicular is the last foot bone to fully calcify. And it's located between the anklebone and 3 cuneiforms.

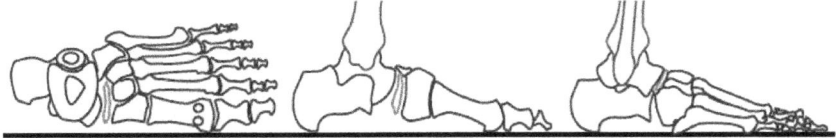

When the tarsal joint falls with each step, this still-growing and still-soft navicular gets jammed in between the already calcified anklebone and 3

cuneiforms. This constant jamming can hinder blood circulation and not allow enough space to grow. All this can interfere with its normal development. As a result, the navicular bone may end up much thinner, weaker, and more fragile. If children frequently jump up and down, this navicular can be even break apart.

Sever's Disease

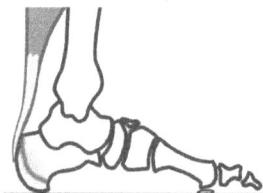

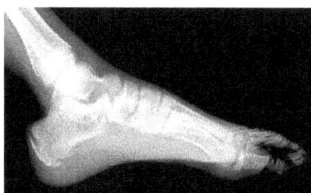

 This is an inflammation of the growth plate located at the back of the heel bone. When the tarsal joint falls, the heel bone tilts. This twists and pulls, stressing the Achilles tendon that is imbedded close to the growth plate. Sometimes this pulling of the Achilles tendon can pull the growth plate apart, causing inflammation in the growth plate and pain at the heel area.

Notes

Chapter 6

Kid's Footprints

The footprints from Harris Mat foot imprinter show how the weight affected the bottom of the feet much more realistically than any present computer images. the print in the arch area indicates the fallen tarsal joint, and dark spots indicate the flattening of the soft tissues. Both footprints are different because both tarsal joints fall differently.

Footprint Analysis

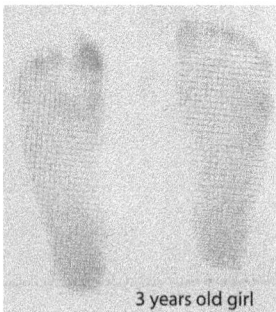

3 years old girl

These 3-year-old girl's footprints show that her right foot wider than the left. The left second toe completely missing indicates the second toe is up in the air—meaning severe collapse of the second metatarsal bone. The light print of her right second toe indicates that this toe slightly up in the air also.

The second metatarsal bone belongs to the centerline of the foot—the highest part of the arch. When the arch falls through the centerline of the foot, the second toe that attach to the second metatarsal bone goes up the most, and though it instinctively tries to grab the ground, it won't be able to reach to the ground.

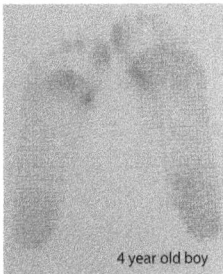

4 year old boy

These footprints of 4-year-old boy with slight pigeon toeing show the right 3 small toes and left 2 small toes barely touching the ground. There are a few dark spots in the left ball of the foot area and one dark spot in the right side, indicating the flattening of soft tissues.

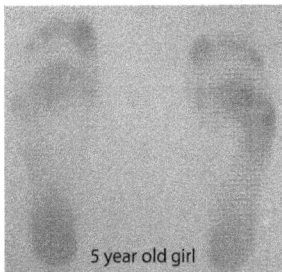

5 year old girl

These 5-year-old footprints missing both pinky toes, and right second toe barely touching the ground. The left tarsal joint fell more forward, making the foot longer, and the right foot fell more laterally, flattening the lateral arch more. The dark spot at the outside ball of the right foot indicates flattening of the soft tissues.

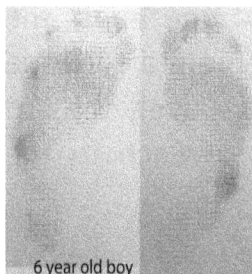

6 year old boy

These 6-year-old boy footprints show total collapse of both lateral arches flattening the 5th metatarsal root on the floor to the point of flattening the muscles under them. And the irregular toe spacing means his foot bones are severely out of alignment.

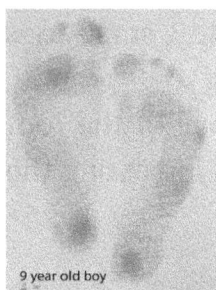

9 year old boy

These are 9-year-old boy footprints. Both pinky toes all up in the air, dark spots at both heels, and the balls of the foot indicates flattening the soft tissues. These dark spots should not be seen even in 70-year-old footprints..!

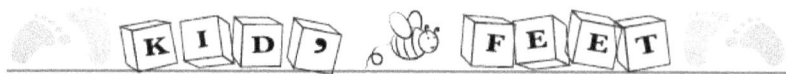

K I D ' S   F E E T

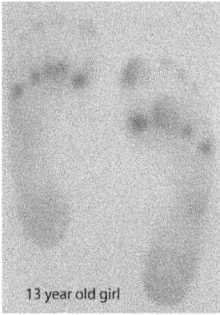
13 year old girl

These are 13-year-old footprints. The dark spots in the ball of the foot areas indicate severely flattened soft tissues under every metatarsal head. Both pinky toes are up in the air.

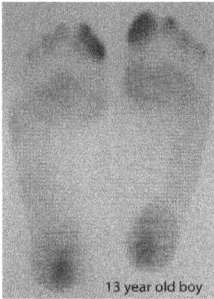
13 year old boy

These footprints of a 13-year-old boy show flattened fatty tissues in the heels, and the left big toes developing callus, and the left pinky toe is in the air. And the left 3rd toe starts to develop into a hammertoe.

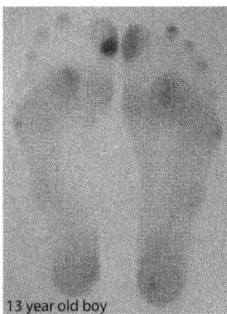
13 year old boy

Another footprints of a 13 years old boy who looks like very active teenager with long toes look like an old man's footprints. The left big toe side developing callus. His right tarsal joints fell more through the centerline of the foot, and both feet look like developing Morton toes (condition of 2nd toe longer than the big toe).

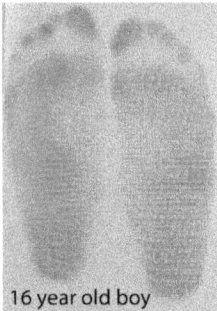

16 year old boy

These footprints of a 16-year-old boy with both his tarsal joints fell completely to the ground—making them flat feet. He's born with flexible muscles. His left 2nd toe slightly in the air.

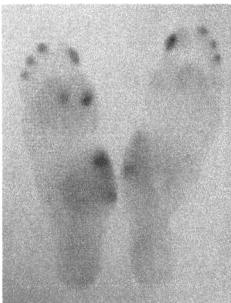

No, these are NOT kid's footprints. These footprints belong to a man in his 50s with his tarsal joint severely fell medially. His navicular and medial cuneiform that form the high medial arch collapsed to the ground to the point of flattening the thick plantar muscles under them. Both pinky toes are up in the air, and in the left foot shows flattening of the fatty tissues under the 1st and 2nd metatarsal heads. If the above 16-year-old boy keeps walking without the orthotics, his footprints can end up like these when he gets old.

All the above footprints are not just indicating the foot problems, they are also telling us the rest of the body moving out of alignment keep damaging all the weight-bearing joints. Just using proper orthotics that align the anklebones can prevent and improve the problems of the fallen tarsal joints.

Notes

Chapter 7

Tarsal Joint & Posture

In This Chapter

- Major Joint Problems
- patella Dislocation
- Leg Length discrepancy
- Scoliosis
- Tilted Shoulder & Face
- Poor Posture
- Bulging Knees
- Fatigue
- Brace Alone
- Pain Killer
- Think about This

Once understand the foot structure and how the weight falls on it, it's easy to analyze how all the problems mentioned in previous chapters and in this chapter are developing from the fallen tarsal joint. It's like analyzing the problems of an automobile running with tilted wheels, or air leaking tires.

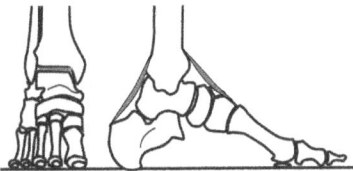

With proper orthotics, we can keep our foot bones and major joints in alignment. As a result, all the ligaments and tendons in and around the foot and major joints can function properly without pulling or twisting.

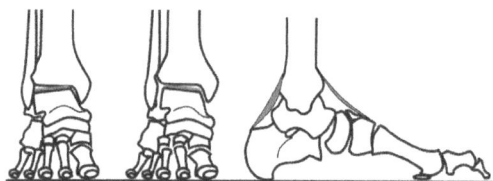 Without proper orthotics, the tarsal joint falls—most cases laterally (outward), tilting the anklebone. Then all the ligaments and tendons in and around the foot and major joints are forced to pull into wrong directions— weakening the joints. This makes the body vulnerable to injuries. In order to stand straight on the fallen tarsal joint, the leg has to stand on the back part of the anklebone—stretching the ligaments and tendons in front of the ankle joint.

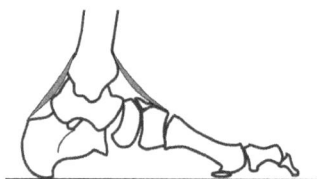 When the tarsal joint falls severely, the ligaments in front of the ankle joint won't be able to overstretch anymore, then the body starts to bend forward—as we see often in elderly people.

Major Joint Problems

The function of the tarsal joint, as the foundation of our body, is weight bearing and the alignment of the entire body structure. This means the tarsal joint should not fall by any weight—just like any other foundation. When it falls, it affects the major joint health, thus, the posture, and hinders growing children's normal growth.

Weak Ankle Joint:

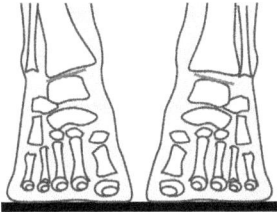 The fallen tarsal joints tilt the anklebones. This makes the ankle joint vulnerable to injuries. Using proper orthotics can even protect ankle joint from straining even on the uneven ground. Even though we hurt the ankle joint for whatever the reason, using orthotics help the joint to heal properly in alignment.

Weak Knee Joint:

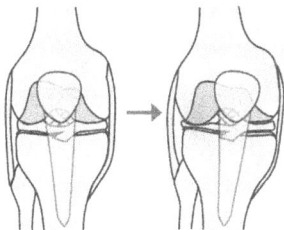 The tilted anklebone misaligns the knee joint. This stresses the ligaments in and around the knee joint: the collateral ligaments, meniscus, cruciate ligaments, and patella ligament. This can cause inflammation and pain in the knee joint and hindering normal growth.

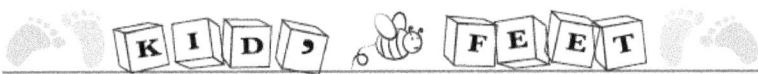

Patella Dislocation

When kids are running and jumping around a lot, the tarsal joint can fall severely worsening the alignment of the knee joints; this can dislocate the patella by pulling off from the center of the knee joint.

Leg Length Discrepancy

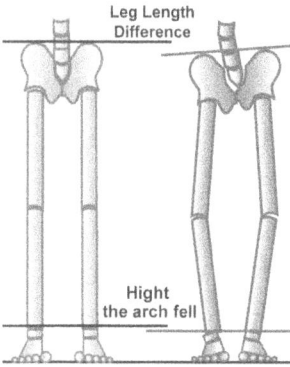

Leg Length
Difference

Hight
the arch fell

Most people, young or old, have one leg shorter than the other, due to differently tilted anklebones, which is from differently fallen tarsal joints. And even 1/8" different arch height with differently tilted anklebones can make 1" different leg length. Because the leg, thigh, and hip bones standing out of alignment shortens the leg length much more than the arch height difference.

Different leg length makes people to limp, a sure sign of their body moving out of alignment. Also, leg length should be measured while standing—from the ground to the top of the hip bone (iliac crest)—not in a lying down posture.

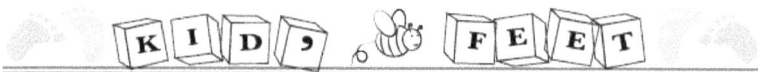

Tilted Hip Joint

Different leg length tilts the hip bones, usually, in a diagonal manner; forward and sideways. This stresses the ligaments and tendons in and around the hip joints by overstretching and twisting—eventually weakens them, and this also can contribute to hernia.

Scoliosis

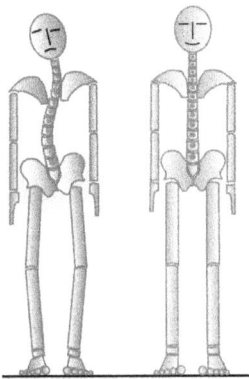

On tilted hips, the spine can only stand with an abnormal curvature, which known as scoliosis. Because the hips usual tilt in a diagonal manner, the spine goes out of alignment from both the front and side view while the vertebrae rotate.

Tilted Shoulder & Face

The tilted spine tilts the shoulder line and the face. The vertebrae rotation makes one shoulder blade higher than the other, pulling and twisting the ligaments and tendons in and around the shoulder and neck joints. In addition, the tilted face stresses the temporal mandibular joints (TMJ) as they are pulled down by gravity while they are tilted.

Poor Posture

All the above problems of the fallen tarsal joint contribute to poor postures. In addition, when children carry backpacks, their bodies must compensate even more, which further worsens their posture.

Bulging Knees

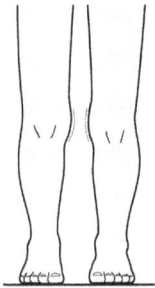

Many children have knees that bulge out on the medial side. Even though their knees may look straight, they are mostly standing out of alignment because of their tilted anklebones. The anklebones typical lateral tilt makes the leg bones stand with lateral tilt, then the thigh bones stand with medial tilt—to stay with the hip joints. This compresses the medial side of the knee joint, stressing the medial side of the joint far more than the lateral side.

This makes the ligaments and other soft tissues on the medial side to sag, while overstretching the ligaments on the lateral side. Standing with this condition stresses the medial side of the joint and slowly damaging the joint. When inflammation happens, the swelling fills the sagging area and causing the noticeable bulge there.

Fatigue

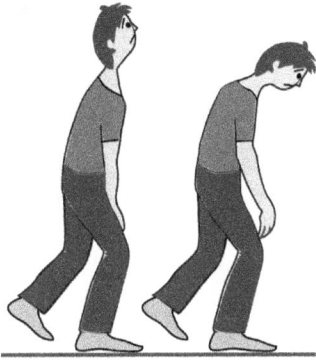

Even though most kids don't express tiredness, their body moving out of alignment wastes energy quite a bit and can be surprisingly draining. Some children do express fatigue and unwilling to participate in physical activities.

Brace Alone

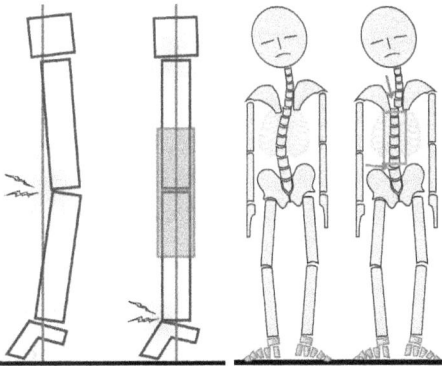

Using braces to align any joint—without aligning the anklebones first—can actually worsen the alignment of nearby joints. Also, when the brace is removed, the joint tends to go back to its previous position.

"Duh..!" was the expression of a mother who had done that to her daughter's scoliosis—after realizing the anklebones have to be aligned first to correct the scoliosis properly.

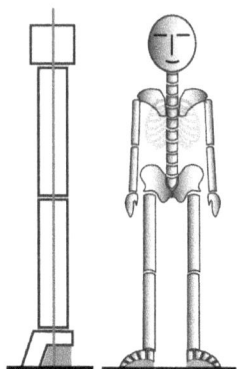

Understanding the structure of the foot and how our body stands on it makes clear why supporting the tarsal joints—to the point of aligning the anklebones—with proper orthotics should be the first step before any treatment.

Pain Killers

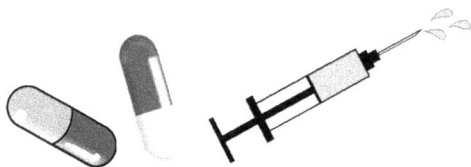

A body moving out of alignment eventually causes mechanical damage and causes pain—sooner or later. Yet, this mechanically caused pain is often treated chemically with painkillers (actually they are nerve killers). As a result, the body deteriorates, both mechanically and chemically at the same time—accelerating the damage.

☆ Think about This

Think about all the activities we do: walking, running, dancing, ice skating, skateboarding, playing ball games, weightlifting, walking on tightropes, etc., etc.

We do all of those on tilted anklebones—and yet, doing so well..!! Truly the human body is an incredible machine.

Now imagine How much more our body can do once our tilted anklebones are properly aligned.

Notes

Chapter 8

Aligning the Anklebones

It may sound so simple that just aligning tilted anklebones at the same height with proper orthotics can prevent and improve all the problems discussed in the previous chapters. And yes, there is one more essential step after aligning the anklebones: standing and walking correctly. We can see the aligning anklebones is the mechanical solution, standing and walking correctly is the software solution. Both must work together to prevent and improve all those foot and major joint issues.

Orthotics, Shoes, & Socks

We know that the things underneath control the alignment of the things above. So aligning anklebones involves everything that goes under our feet: orthotics, shoes, shocks, cushions. Is there anything else?

Yes, the ground we are standing on. They are not perfectly level or aligned, and we have no control over road and terrain condition.

That is why aligning anklebones are even more important. Because when our anklebones are aligned, our body moves with true physical balance. As a result, we can walk and run maneuvering over all different road and terrains with solid balance and confidence—just like automobiles.

We drive our vehicles over all kinds of road or terrains with all different conditions. When the vehicle is properly aligned, it can maneuver over those road without unnecessary damage.

But when a vehicle is not properly aligned, even driving on the normal roads damages the vehicle. On rough roads, the vehicle will get a lot more damage.

Also, for easy understanding, we can compare pedorthic practice to the optometry practice most of us are familiar with. Comparing orthotics to lenses, shoes to eyeglass frames, socks and cushions to coatings on the lenses, and Anklebone Alignment test to vision test.

Orthotics
Aligning anklebones requires extremely precise orthotics, because the surface area on top of the anklebone where our entire body weight falls is only

about one square inch. This means the work demands a high level of skill and accuracy.

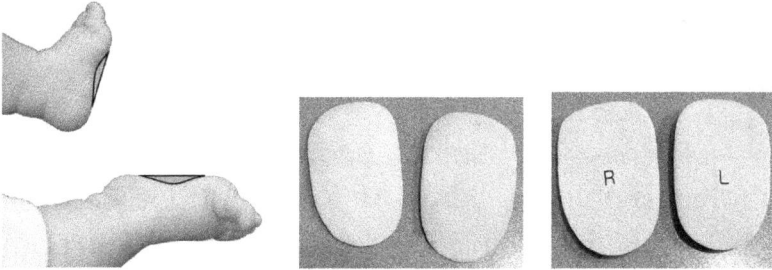

However, for toddlers, simple cookie shape orthotics that fit under their small arches can allow their foot bone to grow in alignment. If the orthotics fit well, you can see them walk steadier without falling. Even though they trip over something, their body have better chance to regain their balance, so not fall.

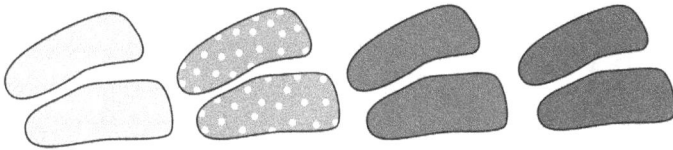

When they reach around 4 years old, the shape of orthotics should be more defined because all the foot bones are present and start to fill in the gaps to articulate the foot joints.

The first step to align the anklebones is finding the proper orthotics.

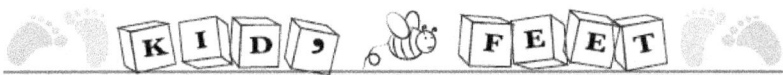

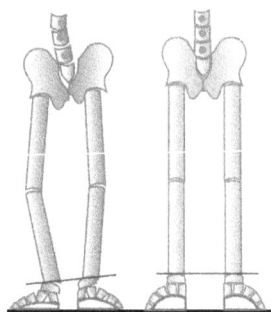

Some people think that the orthotics should be different for each foot because each tarsal joint fell differently. But to bring both anklebones to the same height, both orthotics must be the same. That is why when wearing the orthotics, the foot with more fallen tarsal joint feels more support than the other foot. It's like both eyeglass lenses should provide 20/20 vision.

Shoes

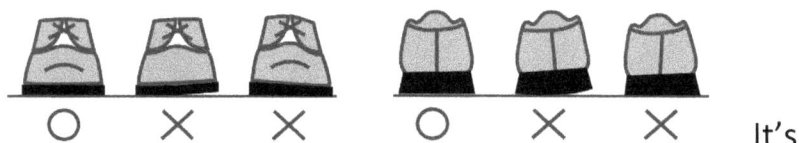

It's important to know there are shoes with tilted bottoms sideways. Using orthotics in those shoes tilt the anklebones again. Shoes with tilted bottoms are like tilted eyeglass frames.

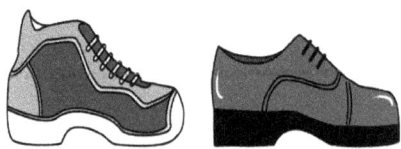

It's better to wear shoes with a little higher heels, as they definitely put the body weight on the arch, where it is designed to handle tremendous weight, or at least the same height front and back. But never use negative heel shoes, the heel lower than the front, because they put the body weight more on the heels—this also throws off the physical balance.

Socks and Cushions

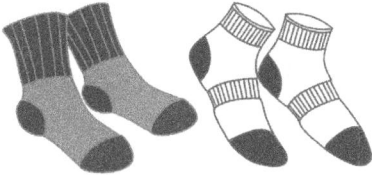

Socks and cushions are not mandatory to align anklebones. However, If you like to wear socks, the bottom of the socks should be the same thickness throughout. Socks with extra padding under the heel or the ball of the foot, or different knitting pattern at the arch area disrupt the even weight distribution and break the balance. You will be surprised when you fail the Anklebone Alignment Test wearing these socks with the correct orthotics and shoes.

Also, if you like to use cushions over the orthotics, they should be the same thickness throughout and should cover the entire orthotics, and they should lay nicely without any crinkle inside of the shoes. This is like the coatings over the eyeglass lenses have to be same thickness over the entire lenses.

Then how can we know all these things are working together to align our anklebones? By Anklebone Alignment test or AA test for short. They all should make us pass the AA test.

To do the AA test properly, we need to know how to control the compensatory behaviors.

Compensatory Behaviors

On tilted anklebones, our body should fall, but it doesn't. Because our body instinctively compensates to keep the body from falling.

The compensatory behaviors use the energy, stresses the brain and nerves, and the compensating joints deteriorate faster. This is why we don't want this system to be always "on mode." It should only kick in when there is a danger of falling. When there is no danger of falling, the system should be turned off.

But on the tilted anklebones, our body is always in danger of falling. Consequently, this compensatory system is always in a working mode to keep our body from falling—until we lie down or align the anklebones.

The compensatory behaviors can be divided into 2 categories: I named them as primary and secondary compensatory behaviors.

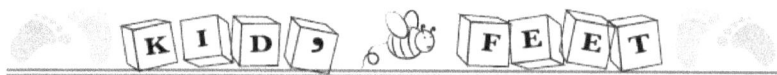

K I D ' FEET

Primary Compensatory Behavior

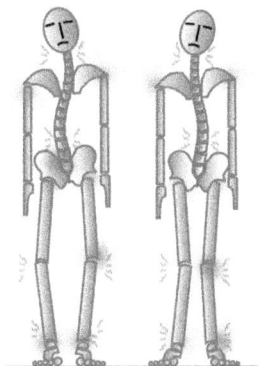

The primary compensatory behavior is our body standing in a zigzag manner. This standing started when toddlers start to learn to stand on the tilted anklebones. Actually, our brain does that instinctively to keep the body from falling. This zigzag standing cannot be controlled by us. It can only be eliminated by aligning both anklebones at the same height with proper orthotics.

When this zigzag standing body needs to lift a weight, it can only lift the weight close to the body.

Secondary Compensatory Behaviors

When this zigzag standing body needs to lift a weight a little away from our body—with extended arms—this body has to compensate additionally to keep the body from falling. There are 3 behaviors: engaging the core (belly) muscles, body tilting (to the opposite direction from the weight being lifted), and toe grabbing. They are deeply programmed on our body and some people don't even know their body acting out these behaviors. I named them as "secondary compensatory behaviors."

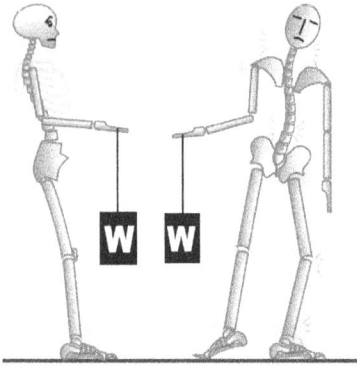

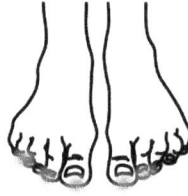

The body tilting and the toe grabbing are happening externally. So, it's easy to detect, and so can be prevented.

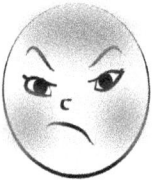

However, engaging the belly muscles happens internally, so it makes hard to detect and only the person can disengage this behavior. One sure sign of this engaging belly muscle behavior is we won't be able to breathe with belly muscles—so we can only breathe with our chest. So, we can control this behavior by being able to breathe with belly muscles.

These behaviors are like squinting of eyes when doing the vision test.

To do the Anklebone Alignment test—our body's physical balance test—these 3 behaviors have to be controlled first. Otherwise, Anklebone Alignment test cannot be done properly.

Anklebone Alignment Test

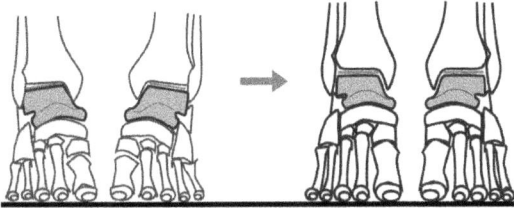

The Anklebone Alignment test (AA test) can verify whether the anklebones are aligned or not.

Onn tilted anklebones, our body cannot use its full strength and its full range of motion. On aligned anklebones, our body can use its full strength and its full range of motion without compensating."

So the AA test is done by while standing lifting a weight that takes an effort to measure the strength with an extended arm(s) to measure the range of motion without compensating; no engaging the belly muscles, no body tilting, no toe grabbing.

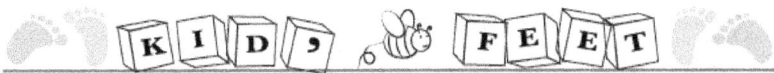

AA Test for One Foot at a Time

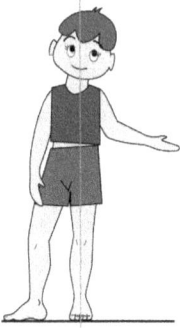

Tell your child to stand on one foot that to be tested, putting their entire body weight on it. The other foot should just stay on the ground without any weight on it.

Their head should be in line with the foot. Extend the arm to position the elbow about 3"-5" away from the body with the hand about 5" lower than the elbow with the palm up.

Tell the child not to tilt their body to the other side of the foot to be tested. Because that shifts the body weight to the other foot and not to use their belly muscles. Tell them just use the arm muscles to resist the pressure you are going to apply onto their palm.

Then, you slowly press down on the kid's heel of the palm to the gravity direction and tell them to resist your pressure. This makes the kid lifting a weight.

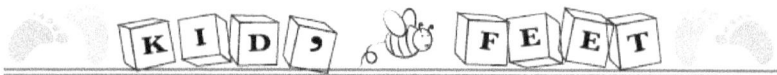

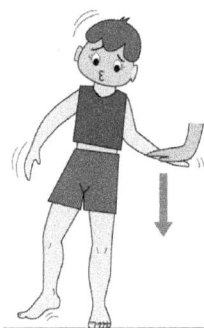

If their anklebone is tilted, their body falls, not being able to use the strength.

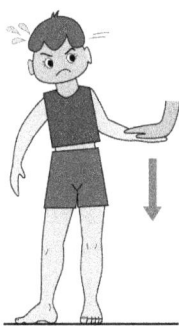

If the kid resists the weight without the orthotics, the kid is definitely compensating. Most likely using core muscles and tilting his body. On the tilted anklebone, no one can utilize their muscle strength unless they compensate.

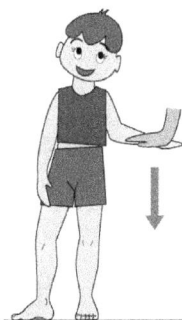

Do the test with orthotics under their arches. If the orthotics align their anklebones, they can use their strength and resist your pressure without falling or compensating. If the orthotics are not aligning, they will fall, not being able to resist.

AA Test for Both Feet

To do the AA test for both feet together, we need to know how to stand on the arch.

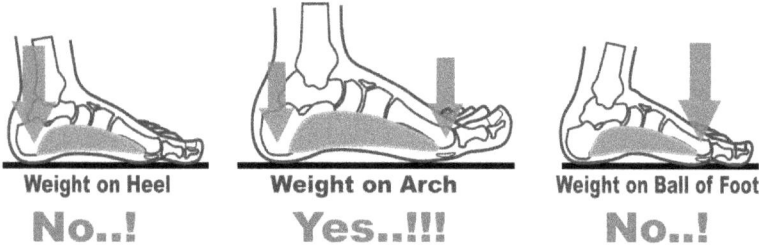

Weight on Heel	Weight on Arch	Weight on Ball of Foot
No..!	**Yes..!!!**	**No..!**

Anatomically, our body stands on the arch. However, mechanically, our body can stand on the heel, ball of the foot, or even on toes. Simply way to know you are standing on the arch is that if we cannot move the heel and ball of the foot, we are standing on the arch.

We can find this spot by moving the hip slightly back and forth. While standing move the hip slightly backward; then you can move the ball of the foot side by side. This means you are standing on your heel; the AA test cannot be done. From there move your hip slightly forward; then the body weight moves forward to the ball of the foot and you won't be able to move neither the heel nor the ball of the foot. This is when you are standing on the arch, and the AA test can be done with this standing. From there, if you move your hip slightly more forward, you can move the heel sideways, that means you are standing on the ball of the foot; the AA test cannot be done.

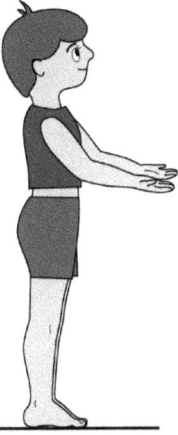

After standing on the arch, lift both hands slightly lower than the elbow in front of the body with elbows 3"- 5" front of the body.

And hold a bar with each hand at each end of the bar. And a person presses down on the middle of the bar to the gravity direction, and tell the kid to resist; then the weight will go all the way down to the anklebones—passing through the standing body.

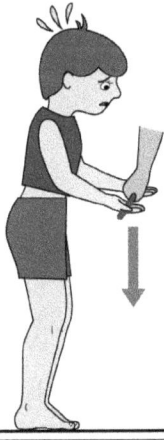

If the anklebones are tilted, the kid unable to utilize his/her muscle strength and his body will fall—unless he compensates.

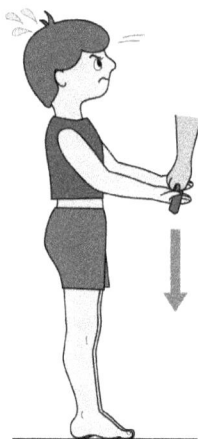

If the kid resists the weight without the orthotics, the kid is definitely compensating. Most likely using all 3 secondary compensatory behaviors: using his core muscles, tilting his body putting his weight on the heel, and grabbing his toes. On the tilted anklebone, no one can utilize their muscle strength unless they compensate.

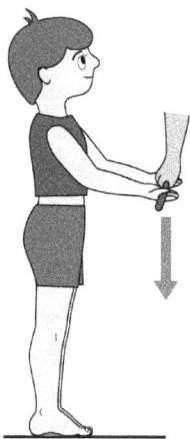

If the anklebones are aligned with proper orthotics, the kid can resist the weight without compensating or falling—while standing on the arch.

Yes, it sounds all so new to most of people, but it's rather a simple test; just lifting a weight with extended arm(s) without compensating: no tightening belly muscles, no body tilting, and no toe grabbing.

If you compensate with the orthotics that algin your anklebones, the same weight becomes heavier, because compensating uses the energy also. This makes you do the 2 tasks at the same time; lifting and compensating. After aligning your anklebones, you can lift the same weight much easier. Using proper orthotics, you can experiment this difference by lifting a weight with and without compensating.

After finding proper orthotics, put them into shoes and do the AA test again to make sure the shoe bottoms are all leveled.

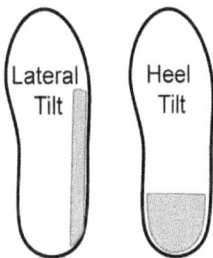

If you fail the AA test, that means the shoes have tilted bottoms, mostly to the lateral side, and very few tilt to the heel side, which means the heel is lower than the front.

Laterally tilted shoe bottoms tilt by 1 post card thickness (less than 1/2 millimeter) to 3 post card thickness (less than 1 millimeter). That's it. And they usually tilt laterally, to the pinky toe side. These shoe bottoms can be leveled by adding correct number of strips (of 2cm wide and 1cm longer than the orthotics length) to the lower inside the shoes.

To find correct number of strips, put 1 strip under each lateral side of the shoes, and do the AA test. Still failed the AA test? Then add another strip and do the AA test again. Still failed the test? Then add another strip, now all 3 layers. That's it. You will be able to find correct number of strips to level the shoe bottoms that tilted sideways. Then attach the correct number of strips inside the shoes on the outside of the shoes.

For the shoes with lower heels can be fixed by adding at least 2 mm thickness pads on the heel areas.

Some shoes are twisted. Those twist shoes make you fail the AA test. Once you twist those shoes properly back, you will pass the AA test.

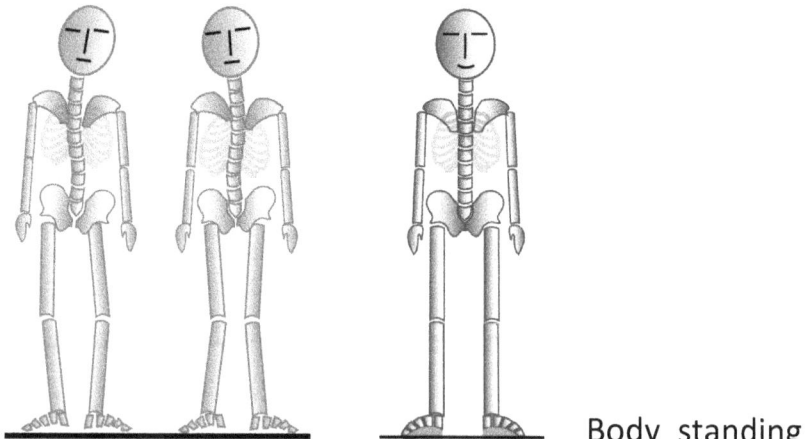

Body standing out of alignment can stand in alignment only after aligning the tilted anklebones at the same height.

Stand & Walk Correctly

Once we align our anklebones, we can finally stand and walk correctly. This means even after align the anklebones with proper orthotics, we can still stand and walk incorrectly, because of old habit of walking incorrectly.

However, toddlers already have a keen sense of balance. That's why with proper orthotics, most of them would instinctively stand and walk correctly.

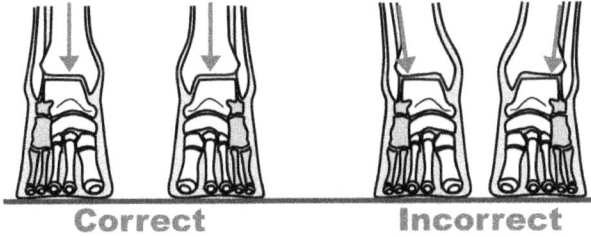

Correct   **Incorrect**   Standing correctly means standing with our body weight straight down onto the anklebones. This makes the body weight to fall on the medial arch.

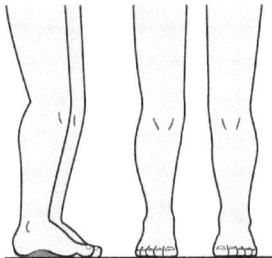

With proper orthotics, we can stand with more comfort. How? While standing with both feet shoulder width apart and slightly bend the knees while slightly pulling them together. This make the body weight to fall where the thickest muscle is located. So blood circulates better at the bottom of the foot. But standing this way without orthotics makes the medial arch to fall more severely.

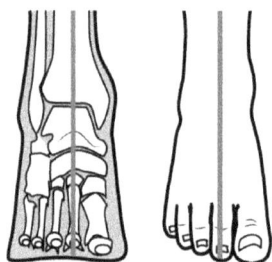 Walking correctly means passing our body weight through the high medial arch when making a step.

If children have a habit of standing and walking with their weight on the lateral side—in attempt to keep the high medial arch from severe falling—they need to move their body weight from the lateral arch to the medial arch. With proper orthotics, their arches not going to fall anymore.

Also, developing a sense at the bottom of the foot as to where the body weight falls, and keep the body weight on the medial arch, we can soon make a habit of standing and walking correctly.

If they keep walking on the outside of the foot, the outside of their shoes will wear down. This tilts the anklebones again. However, the good news is that when the anklebones tilt because of the tilted shoe bottoms while using proper orthotics, our body send out a signal with pain before significant damage happens, because with proper orthotics, the tarsal joint would not compensate.

Then all we need to do is level the shoe bottoms, then pain disappears instantly—it's like a pain from a tilted joint instantly goes away when the joint is released back to its alignment.

Of course, the body cannot stand and walk correctly at all times, because time to time, we need to stand and walk shifting our body weight out of medial arch. But you don't want to stand incorrectly for a long time. Whenever possible, standing and walking correctly prevents problems from doing them incorrectly.

Now, by aligning their anklebones, we can finally let our children to grow in alignment from the feet up and do all the activities with the true physical balance that is coming from alignment, not by compensation.

Whew..!! This is what I discovered so far...

Notes

Afterword

The definition of the word "foot" from the Internet dictionary states simply as the "lower extremity of the leg below the ankle on which a person stands or walks."

The above statements indicate that the foot is the foundation of our body, which means if the foot, the foundation, goes out of alignment, it causes the problems throughout the body. Yet, no one talks about how human foot is constructed with the "TARSAL JOINT." What's more is no one seems to realize this Tarsal Joint in need of support from under to keep the joint from falling.

The foot moves constantly up and down carrying our moving body structure on it. This makes the small foot a moving foundation with relatively tall and heavy moving structure—quite a tricky and heavy task.

Yet, most of us take our feet for granted and don't pay attention until they scream with pain—not knowing most feet and major joint problems, including arthritis and even scoliosis stem from tilted anklebones. It's like driving a car with tilted wheels.

Our foot health is deeply related to our body's well-being; from the way we walk to our frowning faces from foot-related problems. Yet, no one really talks about the matter at hand. When I realized how fundamental it is for our body health, I had to look into the "Instruction from the Manufacturer of the Human Body Machine—the Bible," thinking it would be unfair if this issue were not addressed in it. And it's always exciting to discover helpful information about the well-being of our life from "the Instruction."

I frantically leafed through the Instruction and... I found it..! Of course, in the perfect place...!! Right after it says in the book of Hebrew chapter 12, verse11–12, "^{11}No discipline seems pleasant at the time, but **painful**. However, later on, it produces a harvest of righteousness and peace for those who have been trained by it, ^{12}therefore **strengthen your feeble arms and weak knees,**" and next verse 13 addresses the matter quite clearly in just one sentence..!

"^{13}**Make level paths for your feet**, so that the lame may **not be disabled**, but rather **be healed**." (NIV)

Another translation reads:

"**Make straight paths for your feet**, so that what is Lame may **not be put out of joint** but rather **be healed**." (ESV)

If I decipher this passage correctly, the unleveled path for the feet makes people limp (the lame) and eventually may make them disabled or put them out of joint. To avoid these, we need to make level paths or straight paths for our "Feet."

Once we understand the foot structure with the "Tarsal Joint" that forms the arch, the "leveled" or "straight" paths in these verses should not be interpreted literally as leveled or straight grounds. Because they definitely make the tarsal Joint to fall and tilt the anklebones—misaligning our entire body structure from the feet up and make us lame, eventually may disabling us—with pain.

So, the "leveled" or "straight" paths for our feet should be the paths that maintain *the* proper level and alignment of the foot structure—especially, the anklebones where our body stands.

Also, this passage from the "Instruction" definitely implies that the limping is related to the feet, which makes sense, since the foot is the foundation of our body. However, people think they limp because their hip or back problems—a few of the symptoms of the tilted anklebones.

I was expecting to find this info in the Old Instruction. But it was in the New Instruction. Later, I found why. The time when this Hebrews Instruction was written was when Romans were laying flat stones for the chariot wheels. And our body Manufacturer knew the tarsal joint would fall on those flat stones causing a great deal of damage on our body machine. So He instructed us to make level paths for our feet—not just level paths for the chariot wheels—which can be done by supporting our arch with some materials. That time frame, about 2,000 years ago, there was an evidence that people used some wools in their shoes. I think those people are the ones who built the structures with massive stones that required much strength. However, people were too busy industrializing the world to pay attention to that instruction.

Anyhow, it's astonishing how He addressed the matter in just one sentence; the problems and the solution.

"Most of the fundamental ideas of science are essentially simple, and may, as a rule, be expressed in a language comprehensible to everyone."
(Albert Einstein)

By applying the basic laws of physics, how to keep the Tarsal Joint from falling, the method to test whether the anklebones are aligned or not, and how to walk correctly become essentially simple, and may, as a rule, be expressed in a language comprehensible to everyone. I did my best for now.

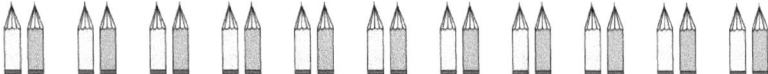

Index

About the Author

When Inna Chon came to the United States from S. Korea in 1982 with a dream and a sketchbook. By 1985, she was working as an animator. For 18 years, her world was images, movement, and imagination rather than words. Then, in 2003, while working as a Disney animator, her trained eyes noticed something that would change the course of her life. As she analyzed walking cycles frame by frame, she was realized people are moving with tilted anklebones. That shocking discovery changed her course of life from doing things for eyes to everything for the feet.

She began talking about what she had discovered, eager to share how important to align their tilted anklebones. But not everyone was ready to listen. Many dismissed her ideas, but Inna couldn't ignore what she knew: people will keep suffering from problems their feet were quietly causing—like her dear oldest sister. She felt a deep conviction that she had to keep speaking until the feet get the proper attention from people.

There was a problem—she needed to master English to tell her story. Learning a new language at 45, surrounded by a Korean-speaking community in S. California, wasn't easy. But in 2015, she moved to Washington State, immersing in English-speaking environments, joined Toastmasters clubs and began to find her voice.

Her persistence, courage, and love of challenge helped her grow—in language and in spirit. She believes each step toward a goal produces the fruits of the Holy Spirit (Galatians 5:22–23), the true tools for harvesting righteousness and peace (Hebrews 12:11), and for living a full and meaningful life.

Now, for over 22 years, still chasing the mystery of the feet with the same passion, she fills her creative side with cooking colorful healthy dishes, designing and altering clothes, playing piano, and gardening.

Now, she's stepping into a new chapter—knocking on doors for speaking opportunities, ready to share her story, her discoveries, and the message she believes can change lives from the feet up.

if any organization or group likes to invite Inna to hear her what she gets to say about the foot, contact her at: innachon2@yahoo.com

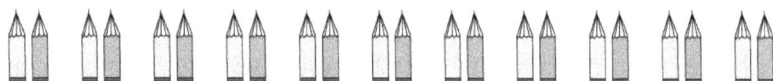

Know the Truth
&
the Truth will Set You Free

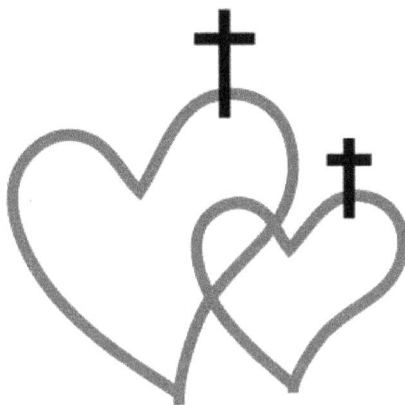

www.ingramcontent.com/pod-product-compliance
Lightning Source LLC
Chambersburg PA
CBHW071136280326

41935CB00010B/1244